A-Z Notes in Radiological Practice and Reporting

Series Editors
Carlo Nicola De Cecco
Andrea Laghi

W0050420

Valeria Panebianco
Jurgen J. Fütterer

MDCT and MRI in Genitourinary Imaging

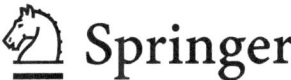 Springer

Valeria Panebianco
Department of Radiological
Science, Oncology and
Pathology
Sapienza University of Rome
Rome
Italy

Jurgen J. Fütterer
Department of Radiology
and Nuclear Medicine
Radboudumc
Nijmegen
The Netherlands

MIRA Institute for Biomedical
Technology and Technical
Medicine
University of Twente
Enschede
The Netherlands

ISBN 978-88-470-5704-3   ISBN 978-88-470-5705-0   (eBook)
DOI 10.1007/978-88-470-5705-0
Springer Milan Heidelberg New York Dordrecht London

Library of Congress Control Number: 2014956379

Printed on acid-free paper

Springer is part of Springer Science+Business Media (www.springer.com)

Foreword to This Series

A-Z *Notes in Radiological Practice and Reporting* is a new series of practical guides dedicated to residents and general radiologists. The series was born thanks to the original idea to bring to the public attention a series of notes collected by doctors and fellows during their clinical activity and attendance at international academic institutions. Those brief notes were critically reviewed, sometimes integrated, cleaned up, and organized in the form of an A-Z glossary to be usable by a third reader.

The ease and speed of consultation and the agility in reading were behind the construction of this series and were the reasons why the booklets are organized alphabetically, primarily according to disease or condition. The number of illustrations has been deliberately reduced and focused only on those ones relevant to the specific entry.

Residents and general radiologists will find in these booklets numerous quick answers to frequent questions occurring during radiological practice, which will be useful in daily activity for planning exams and radiological reporting.

Each single entry typically includes a short description of pathological and clinical characteristics, guidance on selection of the most appropriate imaging technique, a schematic review of potential diagnostic clues, and useful tips and tricks.

The series will include the most relevant topics in radiology starting with cardiac imaging and continuing with the gastrointestinal tract, liver, pancreas and bile ducts, and genitourinary apparatus during the first 2 years. More arguments will be covered in the next issues.

The Editors put a lot of their efforts in selecting the most appropriate colleagues willing to exchange with readers their own experiences in their respective fields. The result is a combination of experienced professors, enthusiastic researchers, and young talented radiologists working together within a single framework project with the primary aim of making their knowledge available for residents and general practitioners.

We really do hope that this series can meet the satisfaction of the readers and can help them in their daily radiological practice.

Latina, Italy   Andrea Laghi
                                                        Carlo Nicola De Cecco

Contents

Contributors

Flavio Barchetti Department of Radiological Sciences, Oncology and Pathology, Sapienza University of Rome, Rome, Italy

Giovanni Barchetti Department of Radiological Sciences, Oncology and Pathology, Sapienza University of Rome, Rome, Italy

Maria Giulia Bernieri Department of Radiological Sciences, Oncology and Pathology, Sapienza University of Rome, Rome, Italy

Valerio Forte Department of Radiological Sciences, Oncology and Pathology, Sapienza University of Rome, Rome, Italy

Elena Lucia Indino Department of Radiological Sciences, Oncology and Pathology, Sapienza University of Rome, Rome, Italy

Abbreviations

ACTH	Adreno cortico tropic hormone
APN	Acute pyelonephritis
BOLD	Blood oxygen level-dependant
BPH	Benign prostatic hyperplasia
CIN	Contrast-induced nephropathy
CNR	Contrast-to-noise ratio
CT	Computed tomography
DLP	Dose-length product
DNA	Deoxyribonucleic acid
DTPA	Diethylenetriaminepentaacetic acid
DW	Diffusion–weighted
FIGO	International federation of gynecology and obstetrics
Gd	Gadolinium
hCG	Human chorionic gonadotropin
HPC	Haemangiopericytoma
HPV	Human papilloma virus
HU	Hounsfield unit
IVC	Inferior vena cava
IVP	Intravenous pyelogram
JCT	Juxtaglomerular cell tumor
MR	Magnetic resonance

MRI	Magnetic resonance images
OGCNs	Ovarian germ cell tumors
PFTC	Primary fallopian tube carcinoma
PID	Pelvic inflammatory disease
RCC	Renal cell carcinoma
RT	Radiotherapy
SCr	Serum creatinine
T1W	T1-weighted
T2W	T2-weighted
TCC	Transition cell carcinoma
UE	Ureteral ectopia
US	Ultrasound
UTO	Urinary tract obstruction
VHL	Von Hippel-Lindau
VUR	Vesicoureteral reflux

A

Abscess, Renal and Percutaneous Drainage of Kidney

- Renal abscess is defined as a parenchymal fluid-filled mass of infectious origin containing suppurative material and delineated by a pseudocapsule. It is usually a sequela of acute renal infection, in particular pyelonephritis or bacterial nephritis, and although the inflammatory process is reversible, it can occasionally result in liquefactive necrosis and abscess formation.
- *CT*: CT is the most accurate modality for the detection of renal abscess; it usually appears as a spherical mass with a thick wall; gas may be visible within the collection. After contrast administration, abscess wall enhances, whereas there is no central enhancement ("ring" sign or pseudocapsule) within the parenchyma surrounded by an area of hypoattenuating cortex at the nephrographic phase. Fascial and septal thickening are usually present. MRI: rim enhancement of masses >1 cm. The puncture and drainage of most abscesses can be performed with CT guidance. When the upper pole is involved, CT is indicated to avoid trauma to the spleen or pancreas.

V. Panebianco, J.J. Fütterer, *MDCT and MRI in Genitourinary Imaging*,
A-Z Notes in Radiological Practice and Reporting,
DOI 10.1007/978-88-470-5705-0_1, © Springer-Verlag Italia 2015

- A perinephric abscess may develop directly from acute pyelonephritis, but it can also result from rupture of a renal abscess into the perirenal space or from extension of inflammatory disease outside Gerota's fascia; it can even involve iliopsoas muscles and extend to the pelvis.

Abscess, Prostatic

- Prostate abscess is a closed pocket containing pus within the prostate. Predisposing factors for periprostatic or prostatic abscesses are diabetes mellitus, urethral catheterization or manipulation, and an immunocompromised status. Most abscesses are infected; any portion of the prostate can be involved and it can communicate with the urethra.
- CT: CT can detect a prostatic abscess (single or multilocular area of low attenuation). Once diagnosed, it can be drained using endorectal US guidance, and a perineal or transurethral drainage approach can be used.
- MRI: MR imaging is usually not performed for this condition, an abscess should be suspected when a cystic lesion with thickened walls, septa, or heterogeneous contents is seen in a patient with typical clinical finding T1W can show enlargement with or without a decrease in signal intensity. On T2W images, the abscess shows higher signal intensity than the adjacent peripheral zone. The postcontrast acquisition can show a typical peripheral strong enhancement.

Abscess, Tubo-ovarian

- It is the term for a variety of infections that involve the fallopian tubes, the ovaries, and the surrounding tissues and often originates from pelvic inflammatory disease; other causes, less frequent, can be Crohn's disease, diverticulitis, perforated appendicitis, and pelvic surgery.

- Symptoms vary in large scale and may be atypical: lower abdominal pain, fever, elevated blood C-reactive protein level, and adnexal tenderness.
- CT: The abscess manifests as bilateral thick-walled, fluid-filled adnexal masses. The abscess wall and adjacent soft tissue inflammation enhance intensely. Internal gas bubbles, which are unusual, are the most specific sign of an abscess.
- MRI: Tubal enlargement can be easily seen on MRI images and is characterized by the tortuous folding of fluid-filled structures on T2-weighted images. Associated findings include thickening of the uterosacral ligaments, infiltration of the presacral fat secondary to edema, hydronephrosis, and indistinct margins of adjacent bowel loops.
- Treatment classically consists of antibiotics or surgery (such as laparoscopy or laparotomy with drainage of the abscess, unilateral or bilateral adnexectomy, or hysterectomy).

Adenomyomatosis of the Uterus

- It is a benign disease of the uterus, relatively common in women of reproductive age. It is characterized by the presence of ectopic endometrial tissue (glands and stroma) within the myometrium.
- Most patients present with menorrhagia and dysmenorrhea. Three different forms may be identified: diffuse adenomyosis (most common form), focal adenomyosis/adenomyoma, and cystic adenomyosis.
- MRI: MRI is the modality of choice for the diagnosis, with a very high sensitivity and specificity. On T2W sequences, it is indicated by an irregular thickening of the junctional zone of

the myometrium, often containing some small high T2 signal regions, which correspond to islands of endometrial glands with cystic change or hemorrhage. After administration of contrast, it may show enhancement of the ectopic glands.

- CT: CT is not routinely used as it is unable to diagnose adenomyomatosis.

Adnexal Torsion

- It is an uncommon gynecological emergency, potentially lethal, that may occur in women of any age, but it is more common during reproductive age. It is the result of axial rotation of the ovary and/or the fallopian tube about its vascular pedicle; it is generally unilateral, with a slight right-sided predilection. This condition may be partial or total, and it can be intermittent or maintained. It causes severe lower abdominal and pelvic pain due to arterial and venous stasis; if untreated, the torsed ovary becomes hemorrhagic and often necrotic.
- CT and MRI: CT and MRI may be useful when a sonogram is indeterminate. CT and MRI show an enlarged, usually edematous, or in some cases hemorrhagic ovary, with peripheral follicles; lack of enhancement may be seen. The involved ovary can assume a midline position; other common findings include a small amount of free fluid and engorgement of blood vessels. MRI is not the imaging modality of choice as urgent imaging is required; it demonstrates hyperintensity on both T1W and T2W sequences due to its edematous and hemorrhagic composition.

Agenesis, Renal

- Congenital absence of one (unilateral) or both (bilateral) kidneys. If bilateral (Potter syndrome), the condition is fatal,

whereas if unilateral, patients can have a normal life expectancy and it could be asymptomatic.
- CT and MRI: CT and MRI show the absence of a kidney, with associated hypertrophy of the remaining kidney to compensate. An empty renal fossa does not always mean renal agenesis: it is really important to ensure that the kidney is actually missing (i.e., check for a pelvic ectopic kidney or cross-fused renal ectopia).

Amyloidosis of the Kidneys

- Amyloidosis is a constellation of diseases resulting in the deposition of abnormal protein (amyloid) in various tissues. It can be primary, if associated with monoclonal plasma cell dyscrasias, or secondary, if associated with chronic inflammatory processes (tuberculosis, rheumatoid, arthritis, Crohn's disease, etc.). Lymphoproliferative disorder should be excluded.
- CT and MRI: Imaging findings are not specific. CT and MRI may show enlarged kidneys in acute stages, while in chronic stages, kidneys may appear smaller than normal.

Amyloidosis of the Bladder

- Primary bladder amyloidosis is rare; more often, it is secondary bladder amyloidosis, both presenting with hematuria. The diagnosis is made by histologic examination. Once detected, systemic amyloidosis or a malignant lymphoproliferative disorder should be excluded.
- CT and MRI: It results in a thickened, irregular bladder wall, and the imaging appearance mimics that of an infiltrating neoplasm. Magnetic resonance imaging reveals amyloid infiltration as a hypointense region on T2-weighted images.

Androgenital Syndrome (AGS)

- Also called congenital adrenal hyperplasia, it is an autosomal recessive condition leading to impaired hormone synthesis: cortisol and aldosterone, produced in the adrenal glands. In 95 % of cases, the genetic alteration is to deficiency of the enzyme 21-hydroxylase.
- Clinically, girls and women develop virilization and boys have precocious puberty. In a subject that has a clinical suspicion, the diagnosis of 21-hydroxylase deficiency is done by evaluating the value of baseline plasma 17-OH progesterone (very high in the classical forms) or after ACTH stimulation.
- CT and MRI reveal large adrenals that are cerebriform in outline. Adrenal rest tissue in other locations also enlarges. This condition should be suspected in an infant with enlarged adrenal glands. Acquired adrenogenital syndrome is most often due to an adenoma and less often to an adrenocortical carcinoma.

Angiography, Renal

- It is an x-ray study of blood vessels to the kidney; contrast is injected into a catheter that has been placed into renal blood vessels. It provides diagnostic imaging, and also endovascular therapy can be applied in the same sitting.
- It is performed to evaluate various vascular conditions, such as aneurism and stenosis.

Angiomyolipoma, Renal (AML)

- The most common benign tumor of the kidney. It is composed of abnormal blood vessels, smooth muscle, and fatty components. Angiomyolipomas are strongly associated with a genetic disease called tuberous sclerosis, in which most individuals have several angiomyolipomas affecting both kidneys. They are also commonly found in women with a rare lung disease, lymphangioleiomyomatosis. It is often found incidentally when the kidneys are imaged for other reasons or as part of screening in patients with tuberous sclerosis. Ninety percent are unilateral and single; 10 % are multiple and bilateral. Symptomatic presentation is most frequently with spontaneous retroperitoneal hemorrhage; the risk of bleeding is proportional to the size of the lesion (high risk if >4 cm in diameter).

- The best diagnostic clue consists an intrarenal fat-containing mass, but a proportion of angiomyolipomas are fat-poor (numbers). CT: well-marginated cortical heterogeneous tumor, with a variable amount of fat. Variable enhancement pattern based on the amount of fat and vascular components. Rare calcifications. MRI: variable signal intensity. It shows hyperintensity on T1 sequences, signal loss in fat-suppression sequences, and significant enhancement after contrast administration if the tumor contains high vascular components.

Anterior Pararenal Space

- It is the portion of retroperitoneum that extends between the posterior surface of the parietal peritoneum and the anterior reflection of perirenal fascia. It is bounded laterally by the lateroconal fascia.
- This area contains the pancreas, duodenal loop, retroperitoneal segments of the ascending and descending colon, the roots of the small bowel mesentery, and transverse mesocolon.

- It is difficult to identify on CT/MRI in normal conditions, but it becomes more visible if there is a fluid collection or a disease process; moreover, fluid can separate the two layers of the perirenal fascia and collect behind the kidney. Disease or fluid in the anterior pararenal space usually originates from pancreatitis, perforating/penetrating ulcer, and diverticulitis.

ARPKD and ADPKD

- Autosomal recessive or dominant polycystic kidney disease: An inherited progressive condition that may manifest in different ages and with varying expression, potentially deleterious to renal function.

Arteriovenous Communications

- It is a very uncommon condition; 70–80 % of arteriovenous communications in the kidney are arteriovenous fistulas (AVFs). The most common causes of AVF are penetrating traumas, but it can also be idiopathic or it can be secondary to surgery, tumors, and inflammation, post biopsy.
- The best diagnostic choice is contrast-enhanced CT; these lesions enhance to the same extent as the adjacent aorta, while thrombosed lesions show no contrast enhancement. Visualization of an enlarged feeding renal artery and draining vein confirms the nature of AVF.
- Treatment of choice is embolization of this fistula.

Artifacts

- Artifacts are components of the image that do not reproduce faithfully actual anatomical structures because of addition, deletion, or distortion of information. It is rather common in clinical MR imaging. They can potentially degrade images sufficiently to cause inaccurate diagnosis.
- CT: The most common CT artifacts are as follows: (1) Volume averaging: it is present in every CT image; it occurs when a dense object lying off-center protrudes part of the way into the x-ray beam. (2) Beam hardening: it results from greater attenuation of low-energy x-ray photons than high-energy x-ray photons as they pass through tissue. It produces dark streaks which extend from structures of high x-ray attenuation, such as bone, arms, high-density objects (vascular clips, dental fillings), or contrast. (3) Motion artifact: it is secondary to voluntary or involuntary movements of the patient, such as peristalsis or breathing; it produces dark streaks or organ duplication of the margin. (4) Ring artifact: if one of the detectors is out of calibration, the detector will give an erroneous reading at each angular position, resulting in a circular artifact. In particular, when central detectors are affected, they will create a dark smudge at the center of the image.
- The most common MRI artifacts are as follows: (1) Motion artifact: it can cause ghost image of the moving structures or it can produce blurring of the image. Spin-echo sequences, particularly those with long echo times, are especially sensitive to motion. The most common causes of image degradation due to motion are breathing, peristalsis, and flow-related artifacts. (2) Chemical shift misregistration: when substances of markedly different molecular composition are immediately adjacent to each other, localized image misregistration

occurs at the interface between the two substances, due to different resonant frequencies. It produces a line of high signal intensity on one side of the fat–water interface and a line of signal void at the opposite side of the interface; it can be frequently seen along the bladder wall or renal margins. (3) Magnetic susceptibility artifact: it refers to a distortion in an MR image induced by a metallic object, such as orthopedic devices, surgical clips, and wires. It produces an area of signal void and a distortion of the image close to the metal implant. (4) Aliasing ("wraparound artifact"): it occurs when a body part is larger than the imaging field; those portions outside the field will be projected back upon the primary image.

Ascites

- Ascites means fluid in the peritoneal cavity. Classic ascites is either a transudate or exudate based on total protein concentration. The most common cause of ascites is portal hypertension due to liver disease; other causes are peritoneal carcinomatosis, infections, and conditions leading to hypoalbuminemia. It can also appear in patients with end-stage renal disease, called nephrogenic ascites, probably due to altered peritoneal membrane permeability or impaired resorption secondary to peritoneal lymphatic obstruction.
- CT: Ascitic fluid may enhance on delayed contrast-enhanced CT. MRI: A transudate is hypointense on T1-weighted images and hyperintense on T2-weighted images, whereas an exudate has a higher signal intensity on T1-weighted images than a transudate (explain why! Contents of the fluid).

Suggested Reading

Barrett JF, Keat N. 2004. Artifacts in CT: Recognition and Avoidance1. Radiographics; 24(6):1679–91.

Porter BA, Hastrup W, Richardson ML, et al. 1987. Classification and investigation of artifacts in magnetic resonance imaging. Radiographcs; 7(2):271–87.

Haaga JR, Lanzieri CF, Gilkeson RC. 2002. CT and MR Imaging of the Whole Body. Volume 2, Fourth Edition. Mosby.

Kawashima A, Sandler CM, Goldman SM, et al. 1997. CT of renal inflammatory disease. RadioGraphics;17:851– 866.

Woodward PJ, Kennedy A, Sohaey R, et al. 2011. Diagnostic Imaging-Obstetrics (2th edition) Amirsys.

Brant WE, Helm CA. 2012. Fundamentals of Diagnostic Radiology (4th edition). Wolters Kluwer-Lippincott Williams & Wilkins.

Pusey E, Lufkin RB, Brown RK et al. 1986. Magnetic resonance imaging artifacts: mechanism and clinical significance. Radiographics; 6(5):891–911.

Algaba F. 2008. Renal adenomas: pathological differential diagnosis with malignant tumors. Advances in urology.

Nichols DH, Julian PJ. 1985. Torsion of the adnexa. Clin Obstet Gynecol; 28(2):375–80.

B

Benign Prostatic Hyperplasia

- Benign prostatic hyperplasia (BPH), also called benign hypertrophy or hyperplasia, adenomatous hypertrophy, or simply adenoma, increases with age. Most benign hyperplasia occurs in the transition zone and only occasionally in the periurethral glandular zone. Sporadic BPH can be seen in the peripheral zone. Some enlarged glands contain cysts, calcifications, or even regions of hemorrhage.
- Transrectal US can easily detect benign prostatic hyperplasia; it appears like a heterogeneous mass that dislocates the prostatic peripheral zone.
- Due to poor parenchyma differentiation, CT is not as performed as MRI in evaluating BPH. BPH is hypointense on T1-weighted images and heterogeneous, ranging from hypo- to hyperintense, on T2-weighted images. It is difficult to discriminate between cancer and BPH, even with MR imaging.

Biopsy of the Renal Parenchyma

See section "CT-guided biopsy of the kidney".

V. Panebianco, J.J. Fütterer, *MDCT and MRI in Genitourinary Imaging*,   13
A-Z Notes in Radiological Practice and Reporting,
DOI 10.1007/978-88-470-5705-0_2, © Springer-Verlag Italia 2015

Bladder Carcinoma

- Primary bladder cancer is three times more common in men than women and more common in whites than blacks. Transitional cell carcinoma (TCC) is the most frequent cancer regarding the bladder, followed by adenocarcinoma, squamous cell carcinoma, sarcoma, and small cell carcinoma which are considerably less common and tend to occur in certain settings. Epithelial origin bladder neoplasms are uncommon in the second decade of life and rare in the first. Most bladder neoplasms at these ages are of mesodermal origin.

- The most common clinical presentation is painless hematuria, ranging from gross to microscopic and often intermittent. Ureteral obstruction due to an adjacent cancer is often silent. Spontaneous perforation of a bladder carcinoma is a curiosity.

- CT identifies a soft tissue tumor arising from the bladder wall. Depending on growth, these tumors range from a sessile polyp to bladder wall thickening. In general, CT misses lesions smaller than about 1–2 cm in diameter. Computed tomography also cannot distinguish adherent blood clots from a tumor. CT should be performed using oral and intravenous contrast with thin sections through the bladder with both a 70-s and a 5-min delay. The early images will serve to demonstrate hypervascular areas of the tumor, and the later images are sometimes valuable in outlining the tumor extent along the wall surface. Tumors may be polypoid or sessile and often extend to involve a large area of the bladder wall, including the ureterovesical junction (Fig. 1). Because transitional cell carcinoma is often multifocal, evaluation of the entirety of the urothelial tract should be attempted. Using multidetector CT scans with rapid reformatting, coronal images can be used to check the renal pelves and ureters for the presence of strictures and masses. All images should also

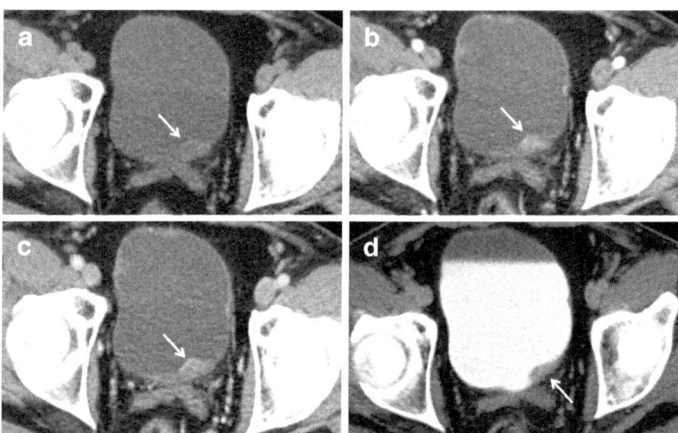

Fig. 1 In basal conditions, CT scans can barely outline a solid mass (*white arrow*) protruding into the bladder (**a**). After intravenous administration of contrast medium, the lesion is well represented both during arterial and venous phase (**b**, **c**). During the urographic phase (**d**), the tumor appears as an image of "minus" compared to the hyperdense bladder which is full of contrast medium

be evaluated for the presence of increased number and size of pelvic and retroperitoneal lymph nodes and distant disease. In cases of advanced disease, CT is probably preferred because of its rapid acquisition and ease of interpretation.

- MRI: Magnetic resonance imaging offers several advantages over other imaging modalities. The multiplanar scanning capability and abundant inherent contrast between perivesical fat, soft tissue of the bladder wall, and urine in the lumen result in excellent contrast resolution. Images should be acquired in at least two orthogonal planes and with high-resolution small fields of view (FOVs). Phased-array surface coils are used to achieve the high resolution necessary for local staging. T1-weighted images are preferred for the depiction of the tumor, invasion into the adjacent fat or

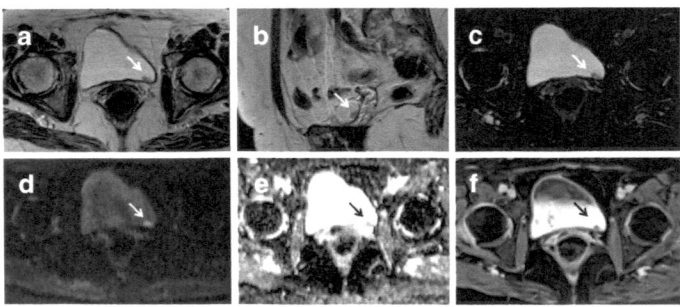

Fig. 2 A hypo-isointense lesion (*white arrow*) located on the left side of the bladder, evaluated in T2-weighted imaging (**a, b**) with also fat signal suppression (**c**). The neoplasm shows a remarkably high value (*white arrow*) in diffusion imaging (**d**) which correlates with low ADC values (**e**), highlighting a tissue with high cellularity (*black arrow*). The mass has no postcontrast enhancement (**f**), showing a hypointense pattern (*black arrow*)

organs, and lymph node and bone marrow involvement. T2-weighted images are used to assess invasion into the bladder muscle, prostate, and seminal vesicles. With injection of gadolinium contrast, carcinomas involving the bladder mucosa and submucosa show early and prominent enhancement. On T2-weighted MRI, the muscular wall of the bladder is of homogeneously dark signal (Fig. 2). Extension into but not through the muscular wall is Stage II disease. Extension of high-signal mass through the wall indicates Stage III disease. Metastasis to a lymph node can be recognized if it leads to nodal enlargement. For local extension, T1-weighted, dynamic, post-Gd-DTPA enhanced images may be of help in delineating a mass from adjacent inflammatory stranding. Coronal images of the upper urinary tract, similar to those with CT or intravenous urography (IVU), can be obtained using a heavily T2-weighted coronal series, obtained either as a volume or comprising multiple slices. MRI shows that carcinomas have a T1-weighted signal intensity similar to that of muscle. T2-weighted images reveal a higher signal intensity than normal bladder wall or fibrosis. Tumor detection is superior with post-Gd-DTPA images, although one should keep in mind that both cystitis and tumors exhibit early MR contrast enhancement. The use of surface coils leads to better image quality than does the use of body coils. Endorectal coils improve visualization of the bladder base and dorsal structures but are of limited use for the rest of the bladder and should not be used. T1-weighted images provide good contrast between hyperintense perivesical fat and isointense bladder wall and detect perivesical fat invasion, spread to lymph nodes, and bone marrow metastases; the latter are identified against the hyperintense normal marrow. T2-weighted images evaluate bladder wall infiltration and prostatic and adjacent structure invasion, although differentiation between tumor and edema is difficult.

Bladder Diverticulum

- Bladder diverticula form when mucosa herniates through overlying muscle. It is uncommon. Diverticula may be primary developmental in origin (Hutch diverticula) or acquired secondary to obstruction and infection or iatrogenic. The latter is more common
- MRI: Bladder diverticulum is well represented using T2-weighted sequences where the diverticula content shows a hyperintense, bladder-like, fluid signal intensity. The diverticulum has a thin wall, in contrast so the native bladder wall which is often thickened as a result of associated bladder outlet obstruction; both possess a low signal intensity on T2-weighted images. The bladder wall, however, may remain its normal thickness in which case a radiological differentiation between a large diverticulum and a bladder duplication is not possible.

- CT: Bladder diverticulum in basal conditions does not own a peculiar aspect that allows to quickly differentiate from the nearby bladder due to similar isodensity and small ones could be skipped on a quick evaluation; performing a Uro-CT is sufficient to detect a pouch filled with iodine contrast medium, which modifies the bladder's profile with a hyperdense "plus" area.

Bladder Exstrophy

- Bladder exstrophy is a rare developmental abnormality that is present at birth (congenital) in which the bladder and related structures are turned inside out.
- Prenatal diagnosis of bladder exstrophy is difficult and sometimes impossible, even using US. Most often, the diagnosis is made after birth with the finding of an exposed bladder.
- Fetal MRI can accurately diagnose a wide variety of urinary tract disorders and must be regarded as a valuable complementary tool to US in the assessment of the urinary system, particularly in cases of inconclusive US findings.

Bladder Fistula

Bladder fistulas are represented by the following:

- *Vesicovaginal fistulas:* These fistulas are correlated to prior gynecologic procedure, obstetrical trauma, adjacent neoplasms, and radiation therapy. Cystography is the procedure of choice to detect these fistulas.
- *Enterovesical fistulas:* These fistulas are the most frequent causes of enterovesical fistulas are sigmoid diverticulitis, colon and bladder malignancies, Crohn's disease, pelvic

radiation, trauma, and infection by actinomycosis, tuberculosis, lymphogranuloma venereum, or an adjacent abscess, such as neglected appendicitis. Indirect signs of a fistula include gas within the bladder and an irregular outline to the bladder wall. A suspected fistula is studied by cystography or barium enema. Computed tomography and MRI outline some bladder fistulas. Gadolinium-enhanced T1-weighted MR images are superior in showing a fistula compared to precontrast images. If a fistula is accessible, contrast injection into the fistula and fistulography or MRI should define it.

- *Uterovesical fistulas:* These fistulas are rare and could be related to prior cesarean sections and may manifest with vaginal urinary leakage.

Bladder, Neurogenic

- Bladder dysfunction is classified into an uninhibited neurogenic bladder, hyperreflexive detrusor (reflex neurogenic, contractile bladder), areflexic detrusor (autonomous neurogenic, flaccid bladder), and sensory or motor paralysis.
- In an uninhibited neurogenic bladder, voluntary external sphincter contraction prevents voiding during uninhibited voiding. As a result, the posterior urethra is dilated to the external sphincter level, and the imaging appearance is similar to a spinning top. These findings occur in infants with an immature bladder and adults with a cerebral cortical lesion (stroke, brain tumor). In infants, the imaging appearance tends to be similar to that seen with posterior urethral valves.
- Patients with a lesion above the lower lumbar level have detrusor hyperreflexia and develop a trabeculated thick-walled bladder. Such a hyperreflexive detrusor is found in patients with multiple sclerosis and lesions inducing spinal cord damage (trauma, tumor, syringomyelia). A large

postvoid residue is common. Bladder contractions result in bladder neck opening, but the striated external sphincter does not open and thus bladder pressure increases. Associated vesicoureteral reflux is common in these patients and, if not corrected, often results in loss of renal function. Lower motor neuron involvement leads to detrusor areflexia. These patients develop a large, thin-walled bladder. No detrusor contractions are evident with an areflexic detrusor. The bladder neck remains open, the external sphincter does not constrict normally, and these patients are incontinent.

- Additional variants of a neurogenic bladder include sensory and motor paralysis. The former is most often found in diabetics. Motor paralysis develops in some multiple sclerosis and polio patients. Urinary incontinence and retention are common problems in multiple sclerosis, often presenting a complex appearance.

Bladder Trauma

- Spontaneous bladder rupture in the absence of trauma is rare but has occurred in a setting of previous radiation therapy, surgery, and infection or is idiopathic. The risk of bladder rupture increases with bladder distention. Perforation of an empty bladder is generally associated with a penetrating injury, either extrinsic or a bone fragment. After blunt pelvic trauma or in a setting of pelvic fractures, bladder or urethral injury is suggested by hematuria or inability to urinate.
- MRI is generally precluded during the immediate post-trauma period by monitoring logistics in a strong magnetic field.
- CT is used to evaluate for pelvic and abdominal trauma. The presence of pelvic fractures and pelvic fluid is associated with bladder rupture, but a bladder perforation cannot be excluded on this study without full bladder distension.

Bone Metastases

- Bone metastases may either be osteoblastic, be osteolytic, or have mixed characteristics. Because bone scintigraphy is sensitive to bone buildup, it visualizes osteoblastic metastases very well and is also sensitive to mixed lesions.

Suggested Reading

1. Anderson J, Carrion R, Ordorica R, et al 1998. Anterior enterocele following cystectomy for intractable interstitial cystitis. J Urol;159: 1868–1870.
2. Kim JK, Park SY, Ahn HJ, et al. 2004. Bladder cancer: analysis of multi-detector row helical CT enhancement pattern and accuracy in tumor detection and perivesical staging. Radiology;231:725–731.
3. Song JH, Francis IR, Platt JF, et al. 2001. Bladder tumor detection at virtual cystoscopy. Radiology;218:95–100.
4. Bernhardt TM, Schmidl H, Philipp C, et al. 2003. Diagnostic potential of virtual cystoscopy of the bladder: MRI vs CT. Preliminary report. Eur Radiol;13:305–312.
5. National Organization of Rare Disorder – Report on Bladder Exstrophy-Epispadias-Cloacal Exstrophy Complex.
6. Szejnfeld PO, Rondon A, Francisco VV, et al. 2012. Prenatal diagnosis of bladder exstrophy by fetal MRI. Jr.J Pediatr Urol. 2013 Feb;9(1):3–6.
7. Beyersdorff D, Taupitz M, Giessing M, et al. 2000. The staging of bladder tumors in MRT: the value of the intravesical application of an iron oxide-containing contrast medium in combination with high-resolution T2- weighted imaging. Rofo Fortschr Geb Rontgenstr Neuen Bildgeb;172:504–508.

C

Claustrophobia

- 20 % of general population have claustrophobia.
- Patient positioning important: Try prone position or head outside the bore or gantry.
- Mild sedation (e.g., benzodiazepine) can be applied.

Cervical Carcinoma

- Cervical epithelium can undergo a series of gradual histologic changes from progressively severe dysplasia to carcinoma in situ (CIS) and invasive carcinoma.
- Invasive carcinoma spreads by direct extension to adjacent organs: vagina, pelvic wall, bladder, and rectum. Metastatic lymphadenopathy occurs commonly in the pelvic lymph nodes, but it also involves the periaortic chains in about 20 % of patients.

V. Panebianco, J.J. Fütterer, *MDCT and MRI in Genitourinary Imaging*,
A-Z Notes in Radiological Practice and Reporting,
DOI 10.1007/978-88-470-5705-0_3, © Springer-Verlag Italia 2015

- The identification of cervical carcinoma in MRI is simple because the high-signal-intensity lesion contrasts with the marked low-signal-intensity cervical stroma on T2W images. Areas of coagulative necrosis may appear as small foci of lower signal intensity within the tumor mass.
- Tumors responding to treatment generally lose signal intensity on T2W images.
- T1W images often doesn't detect smaller lesions because of a lack of contrast between the cervix and tumor.

Cryptorchidism

- The prevalence of undescended testis is 3.5 % at birth and decreases to 0.8 % by 1 year, because many testes descended spontaneously.
- Identification of undescended testis is important because of the increased incidence of infertility and neoplasm if the testis remains undescended.
- If US findings are equivocal or negative and/or a preoperative localization is desired, either CT or MRI can be performed.
- MRI is the best cross-sectional modality to assess cryptorchidism. A disadvantage of MRI in children, compared with CT, is the lack of a contrast agent to opacify bowel loops, which makes detection of the atrophic testis more difficult. Young children require sedation which may be a limiting factor for MR imaging.
- The CT features of an undescended testis are an oval and soft tissue mass located anywhere along the pathway of testicular descent. The accuracy of CT for localization of non-palpable testes exceeds 90 %. Unless it is atrophic or ischemic, the undescended testis has an intermediate signal intensity equal to that of muscle on T1-weighted images and higher than that of subcutaneous fat on T2-weighted images. Coronal T1W images can show gubernaculum testes and spermatic cord,

which can be followed to locate the undescended testes. Diffusion-weighted MRI shows markedly hyperintense testes and helps to differentiate it from surrounding structures.

Cystectomy

- Cystectomy is the surgical removal of the urinary bladder; it is most commonly performed for bladder cancer treatment. After the bladder has been removed, an ileal conduit urinary diversion is necessary. An alternative is to construct a pouch from a section of the ileum or colon, which can act as a form of replacement bladder.
- Because of the complexity of these procedures, early and late postsurgical complications are frequent (including hematoma, urinoma, and abscess); CT is an accurate method for detecting these complications.
- Afterwards, a cutaneous ureterostomy CT allows the accurate depiction of ureters and their surgical anastomoses to the anterior abdominal wall.
- After, an ileal conduit creation multidetector CT allows visualization of the ureters up to the point of anastomosis to the ileal conduit. It is important to evaluate also the enteroenteric anastomosis, most often visible because mechanical suturing is usually performed.
- Subsequently, in continent cutaneous diversion at multidetector CT, the reservoir appears to be partially filled by hypoattenuating material, a characteristic that represents mucous secretions from the bowel.
- Subsequently, an orthotopic bladder replacement multidetector CT allows the identification of a bowel loop in anatomic continuity with the reservoir, a finding that corresponds to the isoperistaltic afferent limb.
- Early complications:

– Adynamic ileus is the most common bowel complication after urinary diversion surgery: it is characterized by dilated loops of small and large bowel with gas–fluid levels and by the absence of a visible cause of obstruction. A CT-based diagnosis of adhesive small bowel obstruction may be made in the presence of an abrupt change in bowel caliber and the absence of another cause of obstruction.

– Fluid collection: The differential diagnosis of postsurgical fluid collections includes urinoma (*see* section "Urinoma"), hematoma, and lymphocele. Unenhanced and nephrographic phase in the presence of hematoma shows a nonenhancing heterogeneous fluid collection. The CT finding of a homogeneous fluid collection with a very thin wall near the surgical clips is suggestive of lymphocele.

Contrast-Induced Nephropathy

• Contrast-induced nephropathy (CIN) is defined as the impairment of renal function; it is measured as either a 25 % increase in serum creatinine (SCr) from baseline or 0.5 mg/dL (44 µmol/L) increase in absolute value, within 48–72 h of intravenous contrast administration. Following contrast exposure, SCr levels peak between 2 and 5 days and usually return to normal in 14 days.

• CIN is one of the leading causes of hospital-acquired acute renal failure. It is associated with a significantly higher risk of inhospital and 1-year mortality, even in patients who do not need dialysis.

Calyceal Diverticulum

• A calyceal diverticulum represents a congenital malformation of the collecting system. These diverticula are usually centrally located within the kidney, adjacent to the pyramids and collecting system. Although most calyceal diverticulum are small (1< cm), occasionally they can be quite large. The incidence of calyceal diverticula is low; the frequency of stone formation within them is high.

- Many calyceal diverticula communicate freely with the collecting system and become opacified during either antegrade or retrograde urography as well as during CT (late phase). Occasionally, the neck of the diverticulum is stenotic, and the diverticulum becomes only faintly opacified or, in some cases, not at all. Detection of faint opacification of a calyceal diverticulum at CT can be assisted by comparing the attenuation within the "cyst" on delayed imaging sequences with the patient first supine and then prone.

Cystitis

- It is the inflammation of the bladder, usually caused by a bladder infection.

   Bladder infections can be caused by inappropriate bladder emptying, damage or irritation around the urethra, and bacteria being transferred from the anus to the urethra.

- Symptoms of cystitis include pain; burning or stinging sensation when urinating; needing to urinate often and urgently but passing only small amounts of urine; urine that's dark, cloudy, or strong smelling; hematuria; and pain low in the belly or in the lower back or abdomen.

- For patients who have frequent episodes of cystitis or in the presence of antibiotic resistance, the possibility of an underlying abnormality should be considered; in such cases, the entire urinary tract should undergo imaging.

- CT scanning is useful when calculus disease, bladder diverticula, colovesical fistula, or perivesical abscess is under consideration.

- In cases of cystitis, MRI findings are nonspecific; the appearance is that of focal or diffuse thickening of the bladder wall. On T2-weighted images, 4 layers of the bladder wall are appreciated. After the intravenous administration of gadolinium-based contrast agent, variable enhancement of the bladder wall is observed. The intensity of enhancement depends on the severity of the inflammatory process.
- MRI is particularly suited for the diagnosis of hemorrhagic cystitis. MRI may demonstrate changes of hemorrhagic cystitis and may permit a determination of disease activity.

Collecting Duct Carcinoma

- Originating from the collecting ducts of the kidney accounts for only 1 % of renal carcinomas. The age of presentation ranges from 16 to 62 years. Collecting duct tumors demonstrate aggressive behavior; a maximum survival of approximately 2 years is reported.
- CT demonstrates renal medullary involvement with an infiltrative appearance and renal sinus encroachment. The reniform contour of the kidney is preserved except when an expansive component is present.
- Collecting duct carcinomas are hypointense on T2-weighted images and hypovascular on angiography. However, there are no specific radiological findings of this entity.
- *Wilms' tumor*: Wilms' tumor represents 87 % of pediatric renal neoplasm. The most common clinical presentation is an enlarging abdominal mass; less common symptoms include abdominal pain, fever, and hematuria. This tumor requires resection and preoperative imaging CT and/or MRI.
- On CT, a Wilms' tumor usually appears as a spherical intrarenal mass, often with a pseudocapsule surrounding it. The tumor is less dense than the normal renal parenchyma on

contrast-enhanced CT scans; areas of attenuation coincide with tumor necrosis, fat deposition, or both. Perinephric tumor extension thickens the renal fascia and obliterates the perinephric fat. Central retroperitoneal adenopathy can be detected by CT. Renal vein and inferior vena caval tumor extension may be shown after an intravenous bolus injection of contrast medium.

- On MRI, Wilms' tumor appears as a large, well-defined mass with relatively distinct margins. It has low signal intensity on T2W images. The tumor often appears heterogeneous on both T1W and T2W images. Currently, CT and MRI appear equivalent for staging Wilms' tumor. However, MRI shows venous extension better than CT.

- *Nephroblastomatosis*: Foci of persistent metanephric tissue are designated as nephrogenic "rests." The presence of multiple nephrogenic rests is termed nephroblastomatosis, which is a precursor lesion to Wilms' tumor. Nephroblastomatosis occurs most often in neonates and is characterized by multiple bilateral subcapsular masses.

- CT is the gold standard. On contrast-enhanced CT, the rests enhanced less than the adjacent normal parenchyma. The hallmark of neoplastic transformation of a benign nephrogenic rest is enlargement on serial CT scans.

- On MRI, nephroblastomatosis tends to be hypointense to renal cortex on T1W images and isointense to cortex on T2W images.

- *Renal sarcoma*: Primary renal sarcomas are rare mesenchymal tumors that often have a poor prognosis. Subtypes of this neoplasm include leiomyosarcoma (the most common renal sarcoma, accounting for about 58 % of all), angiosarcoma, hemangiopericytoma, liposarcoma, rhabdomyosarcoma, fibrosarcoma, and osteosarcoma.

  - Capsular localization, a feature of more than 50 % of these tumors, should suggest the diagnosis on CT. When these neoplasms arise in the renal parenchyma, they are indistinguishable from RCC in CT images. On CT, lipo-sarcoma causes compression without invasion of the renal parenchyma and shows a variety of appearances correlating with their gross and histological features. For example, tumors containing a large amount of mature fat show negative attenuation values and myxoid liposarcoma contains little mature fat, and their predominantly fluid and connective tissue composition results in attenuation values nearer those of water.

CT-Guided Biopsy of the Kidney

- CT is the second-choice modality if the problem is not well seen by ultrasound. The main indication is the presence of a mass of indeterminate nature not identifiable with other methodologies. In most patients, the approach is posterior, with the trajectory chosen to avoid the erector spinal muscle (after anesthetizing locally the renal capsule).
- Cystic masses: Aspirate the fluid and define the thickening of the wall by injecting urographic contrast material. Try to sample, eventually, the solid portion of the mass or the wall thickening. Solid masses: A bolus dynamic scan must be performed to assess vascularity; in case of slightly increased vascularity, aspiration is quite safe.
- The accuracy rate for diagnostic aspiration of renal mass is approximately 100 %. Complications related to such procedures are quite low.

Contrast-to-Noise Ratio

- Relative signal-to-noise differences from two different regions.
- $CNR = (S_1 - S_2)/\sigma$.

- S_1 and S_2 = mean signal intensity from the two regions; σ = standard deviation of the background noise.

Conversion Factors, Radiation Dose

- Estimate of effective dose from the DLP.
- Conversion factor used: European Commission. European guidelines on quality criteria for computed tomography, EUR 16262EN. Luxembourg: Office for Official Publications of the European Communities, 2000. Available at www.drs.dlk/guidelines/ct/quality.
- E_{eff} = Conversion Factor • DLP.

Suggested Reading

Breslow N, Beckwith JB, Ciol M, Sharples K. 1988. Age distribution of Wilm's tumour: Report from the National Wilm's tumor study. Cancer Res, 48:1653–1657.

Kasper HU, Buhtz P, Kruger G, at al. 1997. Bellini duct carcinoma of the kidney-a case report. Gen Diagn Pathol 143:237–241.

Pickhardt PJ. 2001. Collecting duct carcinoma of the kidney: Are imaging findings suggestive of the diagnosis? AJR Am Roentgenol 176:627–633.

Wolverson MK, Houttuin E, Heiberg E, et al. 1983. Comparison of CT with HR real time US in the localization of the impalpable undescended testis. Radiology 146:133–136.

Murphy SW, Barrett BJ, Parfrey PS. 2000. Contrast nephropathy. J Am Soc Nephrol.;11(1):177–82.

Catalá V, Solà M, Samaniego J, et al. 2009. CT Findings in Urinary Diversion after Radical Cystectomy: Postsurgical Anatomy and Complications. Radiographies 29(2):461–76.

Wolverson MK, Jagannadharao B, Sundaram M, et al. 1980. CT localization of impalpable cryptorchid testes. Am J Roentgenol 134:725–729.

Lee JKT, Glazer HS. 1982. CT in the localization of the nonpalpable testis. Urol Clin North Am 9:397–404.

Cushing B, Slovis TL. 1992. Imaging of Wilm's tumor: what's important! Urol Radiol 14:241–251.

Clark, PE; Stein JP, Groshen SG et al. 2005. Radical cystectomy in the elderly: comparison of clinical outcomes between younger and older patients. Cancer 104 (1): 36–43.

Eilenberg SS, Lee JK, Brown J, et al 1990. Renal masses: Evaluation with Gradient echo Gd-DTPA-enhanced dynamic MRI. Radiology 176:333–338.

Friedland JR: GW, Chang P. 1988. The role of imaging in the management of the impalpable undescended testis. AJR Am J Roentgenol 151: 1107–1111.

Uterine cervical carcinoma: comparison of CT and MR findings. Radiology 175:45–51.

Worthington JL, Balfe DM, Lee JKT. 1996. Uterine neoplasm: MR imaging. Radiology 159:725–730.

D

Duplicated Collecting System

- It is one of the most common congenital renal tract abnormalities, characterized by incomplete fusion of the upper and lower pole moieties resulting in complete or incomplete duplication of the collecting system.
- Duplication can be variable: At one end of the spectrum, there is merely duplication of the renal pelvis, draining via a single ureter. At the other extreme, two separate collecting systems drain independently into the bladder or ectopically. Duplex systems may be unilateral or bilateral and can be associated with a variety of other congenital abnormalities of the urinary tract, e.g., ureterocele.
- Most duplicated systems are asymptomatic and diagnosed incidentally. However, where symptoms do occur (infection, reflux, or obstruction), the patient is likely to have completely duplicated ureters. Occasionally, hydronephrosis can be severe enough to result in flank discomfort or even a palpable mass.
- MRI urography may be used as the primary diagnostic method for assessing a duplex ectopic ureter, as well as the

V. Panebianco, J.J. Fütterer, *MDCT and MRI in Genitourinary Imaging*,   33
A-Z Notes in Radiological Practice and Reporting,
DOI 10.1007/978-88-470-5705-0_4, © Springer-Verlag Italia 2015

complications associated with duplex kidneys. Spatial resolution is a limiting factor. MR urography is an extremely useful technique in patients who have the probability of an adverse reaction to radiopaque contrast media.

- CT is able to delineate all these abnormalities, especially when performed during the excretory phase. Maximum intensity projection (MIP) reconstruction software can produce single images of the collecting systems. In an unobstructed system, the diagnosis can be difficult. A duplicated renal collecting system can be suspected by identifying the so-called faceless kidney.

Dilating Uropathy

- Dilated collecting and draining system (ureter, renal pelvis, calyxes): Any condition of the urinary tract that causes or is associated with dilatation of the urinary system. Note that dilatation does not equal to obstruction; obstruction may be one cause for dilatation; other reasons for a dilated urinary tract are laxity, dysplasia, infection, or congenital variations such as megacalicosis.

Dynamic Contrast-Enhanced MR Imaging

- Dynamic contrast-enhanced MR imaging is performed after the administration of intravenous contrast medium to access vascular characteristics of tumors and normal tissues. T1 shortening from contrast agent is considered a measure of tissue perfusion, capillary permeability, and volume of extracellular space.

Suggested Reading

1. Khan AN, Chandramohan M, MacDonald S. 2013. Duplicated Collecting System Imaging. Chief Editor: Eugene C Lin, Sumaira.
2. Croitoru S, Gross M, Barmeir E. 2007. Duplicated ectopic ureter with vaginal insertion: 3D CT urography with i.v. and percutaneous contrast administration. AJR Am J Roentgenol;189 (5): W272-4.
3. Tischkowitz MD, Hodgson SV. 2003. Fanconi anaemia. J. Med. Genet;40 (1): 1–10.
4. Gay SB, Armistead JP, Weber ME et-al. 1991. Left infrarenal region: anatomic variants, pathologic conditions, and diagnostic pitfalls. Radiographics;11 (4): 549–70.

E

Ectopic Kidney

- A renal ectopia is a birth defect in which the developmental of the kidney is characterized by abnormal anatomical location (arrest or exaggeration of normal caudal-to-cranial ascent of the kidney). The incidence is about 1/900 people.
- Patients are most often asymptomatic. Normal pathology can affect ectopic kidneys, but because of the ectopic position, patients could refer nonclassical abdominal pain or urinary disorders.
- Most common associations in patients with renal ectopia are multicystic dysplasia in a fused or unfused crossed kidney, ureterocele, ectopic ureteric orifice, and vesicoureteric reflux (*see vesicoureteric reflux*).
- Ectopic kidney is often an incidental finding at abdominal ultrasonography. Around 50 % remain unrecognized throughout life.
- Contrast-enhanced CT of the abdomen and pelvis shows the abnormalities in patients with renal ectopia.

- MRI shows detailed anatomic position of dysplastic kidneys and eventually ectopic ureteral insertions and/or other associated malformations, in cases where other modalities, which use ionizing radiation or nephrotoxic contrast agents, have failed. One of the disadvantages of MRI includes the need for sedation or general anesthesia in most children.

Ejaculatory Dysfunction, MR of

- MRI with an endorectal coil has been used in man with ejaculatory dysfunction to identify developmental abnormalities of the prostate and seminal vesicles.
- Prostatic cysts along the course of the ejaculatory ducts, seminal vesicle cysts associated with ipsilateral seminal vesicle and renal agenesis, and seminal vesicle calculi can be identified. Evidence of hemorrhage is often seen in the seminal vesicles (short T1 of fluid) in men with hemospermia.
- The normal seminal vesicles measure about 3 cm in length and about 1.5 cm in diameter, with a normal volume of about 13.7 mL. The walls of the seminal vesicles are normally 1–2-mm thick at MR imaging. The ampullae of the vas deferens measure 0.4 cm ± 0.1 in diameter. The ejaculatory ducts measure approximately 4–8 mm in diameter.
- Utricle cysts are pear-shaped structures that, unlike Müllerian duct cysts, do not extend above the base of the prostate. They communicate freely with the prostatic urethra.
- Müllerian duct cysts result from focal failure of regression and focal saccular dilatation of the mesonephric duct. They appear as teardrop-shaped midline cysts extending above the prostate. They do not communicate with the posterior urethra whereas utricle cysts do. These cysts may also cause ejaculatory impairment by obstructing the ejaculatory duct in the midline.

Endometrial Carcinoma

- Cancer of the endometrium is the most common invasive gynecological malignancy in Europe and the United States. The median age of occurrence is 63 years, though 12 % of cases are present in premenopausal women.
- Clinical presentation commonly is a postmenopausal bleeding.
- The most common histological type is endometrioid adeno-carcinoma (75 %); less common types are papillary serous carcinoma, clear cell carcinoma, adenosquamous carcinoma, and undifferentiated carcinoma.
- Staging of endometrial carcinoma is based on the FIGO staging system, which uses a surgical and pathological staging following total abdominal hysterectomy, salpingo-oophorectomy, lymphadenectomy, and peritoneal washings. Tumors are staged on the basis of depth of myometrial invasion.
- US signs of endometrial cancer include heterogeneity and irregular endometrial thickening. Polypoid tumors tend to cause more diffuse and irregular thickening than a polyp and more heterogeneity than endometrial hyperplasia. A uterine fluid collection should raise the concern of underlying malignancy.
- CT is most commonly used to study extent of spread of endo-metrial cancer, but it's necessary to administer oral, rectal, and IV contrast material. CT findings may include the following:

  - Hypoattenuated mass in the region of the endometrial cavity, which may show uniform attenuation or may be heterogeneous, with or without a contrast-enhanced component
  - Polypoid mass surrounded by endometrial fluid

– Heterogeneous soft tissue mass/masses and fluid expanding the endometrial cavity
– Fluid-filled uterine cavity marginated by mural tumor implants

The reported overall accuracy of CT staging ranges from 84 to 88 %.A dedicated pelvic MRI protocol is valuable in the evaluation of endometrial cancer. The imaging protocol consist of using a phased-array coil, administering antiperistaltic agents, using high-resolution sagittal and axial T2-weighted sequences, and using axial T1-weighted spoiled gradient-echo images for lymph nodes study and sagittal T1-weighted spoiled gradient-echo sequences following IV injection of paramagnetic contrast material.

• MRI has proven to be an important tool for the staging of known endometrial carcinoma: MRI can differentiate between superficial and deep-muscle-invasive tumors, such important information for surgical management.
• MR imaging findings may show focal or diffuse endometrioid thickening, which is irregular in thickness, configuration, and mass or widened by polypoid tumor. The signal intensity of the tumor has variable patterns on T1-weighted and T2-weighted images:

– Unenhanced T1-weighted images: Hypo- to isointense to normal endometrium.
– T2: Hyperintense or heterogeneous relative to normal endometrium.
– T1 + (Gd): Carcinoma tissue will enhance less than normal endometrium.

MRI is considered superior to CT for local staging, and post-contrast MRI improves accuracy in detecting the depth of myometrial invasion. If the normal low-signal-intensity junctional zone is intact, myometrial invasion can most likely be excluded.

Endometrial Polyp

- Endometrial polyps are benign small, soft growths on the lining of the uterus.
- They may be single or multiple (20 %), sessile or pedunculated, and much more commonly localized towards the fundal and cornual regions within the uterus. They are most frequently found in patients receiving tamoxifen.
- Endometrial polyps often are asymptomatic although they can be a common cause of postmenopausal bleeding (30 % of cases). In menstruating women, they may cause intermenstrual bleeding, metrorrhagia, and infertility.
- Ultrasound signs of endometrial polyp consist of echogenic, smooth, focal mass in the endometrial canal outlined by fluid.
- Polyps may also be seen at hysterosalpingography as pedunculated filling defects in the uterine cavity.
- Pelvic MRI findings: Endometrial polyps are of intermediate signal intensity on T1W images (but often iso-signal intensity to endometrium) and of low-to-high signal intensity on T2W images; the presence of a central focus of low signal intensity on T2W images indicates a fibrous core, which suggests the diagnosis of an endometrial polyp. Use of contrast enhancement improves lesion detection, but enhancement patterns do not reliably distinguish endometrial carcinoma from other lesions.

Endometrioma

- An endometrioma is a localized form of endometriosis: a benign, estrogen-dependent cyst located outside the uterus, found in women of reproductive age. It usually involves the ovaries and it is bilateral in 1/3 of the cases. Malignant transformation of endometriosis is very rare.

- MRI findings of endometriomas are variable and depend on the concentration of iron and protein in the fluid, products of blood degradation. In fact, the cyst contains altered blood that varies from the usual viscous "chocolate" material to the watery fluid; instead, the wall of these cysts is usually thick and fibrotic, but it may be attenuated. MRI can distinguish endometriomas from most other ovarian masses. It cannot accurately detect superficial implants and adhesions.

On T1W images, MRI of fat-suppressed "chocolate cyst" demonstrates very high signal intensity that becomes relatively hypointense in T2W sequences. This pattern of signal intensities is rarely seen in other masses of any type.

Endometriosis

- Endometriosis is an estrogen-dependent disease classically defined as the presence of functional endometrial tissue outside the uterine cavity and has an estimated prevalence of 5–10 % of women per year. This is distinct from adenomyosis, in which endometrial tissue is confined to the uterine musculature. Endometriosis is divided into superficial and deep and comprises nodules, cysts, and secondary scarring.
- It is mainly found in the abdominal cavity, most commonly on the surface of the ovaries. Less common locations include C-section scars, deep subperitoneal tissues, gastrointestinal tract, bladder, chest, and subcutaneous tissues.
- Endometriosis may be asymptomatic. Common symptom is pelvic pain, including dyspareunia, dysmenorrhea, chronic pelvic pain, urinary symptoms and rectal discomfort, and dyschezia.
- MRI has high sensitivity and specificity for evaluating deep disease and lesion characterization. Lesions usually

demonstrate low to intermediate signal intensity on T2- and T1-weighted images. Typically, the lesions that can be detected with MRI are those that contain degraded blood products and high concentration of protein. T2-shading is the classic MR feature of an endometrioma and is defined as a cystic lesion with hyperintense signal on T1-weighted images that demonstrates T2 shortening resulting in relative hypointensity on T2-weighted images. The cul-de-sac is the most common site of deep pelvic involvement, and the differentiation between normal anatomy and presence of endometriosis in this site is readily made using MRI.

In cases of suspected malignancy, T1- and T1-fatsat sequences before and after the administration of intravenous gadolinium may supplement this protocol.

- Limitations of MRI: Superficial endometriosis (Sampson's syndrome) is most often not visible; nonpigmented lesions will not be hyperintense on T1 and thus harder to detect; small foci may have variable signal intensity; plaque-like implants are difficult to delineate.

Endometritis

- Endometritis refer to an inflammation of the endometrium; it may be acute or chronic. Acute endometritis most commonly occurs in the puerperium and is characterized by the presence of microabscesses or neutrophils within the endometrial glands; chronic endometritis is secondary to the use of intrauterine devices and is distinguished by variable numbers of plasma cells within the endometrial stroma. Cesarean section and multiple vaginal examinations are important risk factors.

- In acute endometritis, symptoms include lower abdominal pain, fever, and abnormal vaginal bleeding or discharge. Chronic disease may be asymptomatic or may occur with intermenstrual bleeding or pain.

  CT plays little role in the diagnosis of endometritis.
- MRI appearance: Uterus with medium signal intensity on T1 and high signal intensity on T2, with loss of the normal uterine zonal anatomy (the uterus can be enlarged). Postcontrast images show intense uniform enhancement because of the hypervascular inflammatory changes and zonal anatomy is not appreciated.

Epididymo-orchitis

- Epididymo-orchitis is the sudden inflammation of the epididymis and testis. It is usually due to infection, most commonly from a urine infection or a sexually transmitted organism. The infection usually begins in the tail of the epididymis and spreads to the body and head. Approximately 20–40 % of cases of epididymitis are associated with orchitis, which is thought to be due to direct extension of infection into the testicular parenchyma.
- Clinical evaluation alone serves to identify most infectious disease affecting the male genitalia, and US is in general the imaging modality of choice. However, MR imaging can be useful as a problem-solving tool when sonographic findings are equivocal.
- At MR imaging, epididymo-orchitis generally demonstrates heterogeneous areas of low signal intensity on T2-weighted images. The epididymis may be enlarged and hyperenhancing on contrast-enhanced T1-weighted images. The testis often demonstrates evidence of orchitis as patchy areas of lower signal intensity on T1-weighted images (inhomogeneous

enhancement). The fluid usually evident in the scrotal sac may outline the bare area of the testis. Visualization of this structure helps to exclude testicular torsion. If fluid within the hydrocele is other than simple fluid (i.e., has very long T1 and T2), the presence of hemorrhage or infection of the fluid is suggested. Gadolinium-enhanced images may be valuable in this regard to demonstrate necrotic or infarcted areas of the testis as nonenhancing areas.

Suggested Reading

Woodward PJ, Sohaey R, Mezzetti TP. Endometriosis: radiologic-pathologic correlation. Radiographics. 21 (1): 193–216. Radiographics (full text) – Pubmed citation.

Bazot M, Darai E, Hourani R et al. Deep pelvic endometriosis: MR imaging for diagnosis and prediction of extension of disease. Radiology. 2004;232 (2): 379–89.doi:10.1148/radiol.2322030762 – Pubmed citation.

Ha HK, Lim YT, Kim HS et al. Diagnosis of pelvic endometriosis: fat-suppressed T1-weighted vs conventional MR images. AJR Am J Roentgenol. 1994;163 (1): 127–31. AJR Am J Roentgenol (abstract) – Pubmed citation.

Zawin M, Mccarthy S, Scoutt L et al. Endometriosis: appearance and detection at MR imaging. Radiology. 1989;171 (3): 693–6. Radiology (abstract) – Pubmed citation.

Sala E, Wakely S, Senior E et al. MRI of malignant neoplasms of the uterine corpus and cervix. AJR Am J Roentgenol. 2007;188 (6): 1577–87. doi:10.2214/AJR.06.1196 – Pubmed citation.

Hardesty LA, Sumkin JH, Hakim C et al. The ability of helical CT to preoperatively stage endometrial carcinoma. AJR Am J Roentgenol. 2001;176 (3): 603–6. AJR Am J Roentgenol (full text) – Pubmed citation.

Davis PC, O'neill MJ, Yoder IC et al. Sonohysterographic findings of endometrial and subendometrial conditions. Radiographics. 22 (4): 803–16. Radiographics (full text) – Pubmed citation.

Schnall MD, Pollack HM, Van Arsdalen K et al: The seminal tract in patients with ejaculatory dysfunction:MR imaging with an endorectal coil. AJR Am J Roentgenol 159:337–341, 1992.

Baker LL, Hajek PC, Burkhard TK, at al: MR imaging of the scrotum:pathological conditions. Radiology 163:93–98, 1987.

"Endometrial cancer: ESMO Clinical Practice Guidelines for diagnosis, treatment and follow-up." G. Plataniotis, M. Castiglione and On behalf of the ESMO Guidelines Working Group.

Hricak H, Finck S, Honda G, Göranson H. MR imaging in the evaluation of benign uterine masses: Value of gadopentetate dimeglumine-enhanced T1-weighted images. AJR Am J Roentgenol.1992;158:1043–1050.

Outwater E, Schiebler ML, Owen RS, Schnall MD. Characterization of hemorrhagic adnexal lesions with MR imaging: blinded reader study. Radiology. Feb 1993;186(2):489–94.

MRI of the Pelvis: A Text Atlas. Hedvig Hricak.

Bauer SB. Anomalies of the upper urinary tract. In: Wein A, ed. Campbell-Walsh Urology. 9th ed. Philadelphia: Saunders Elsevier; 2007: 3269–3304.

Shebel HM, Farg HM, Kolokythas O, El-Diasty T. Cysts of the lower male genitourinary tract: embryologic and anatomic considerations and differential diagnosis. Radiographics. 2013 Jul-Aug;33(4):1125–43.

F

Fistula, Rectovaginal

- Rectovaginal fistulas are rare and represent a small portion of all anorectal fistulas. Enterovaginal and vesicovaginal fistulas are the most common types of complications after radiotherapy of larger gynecologic neoplasms and after surgery. Women with colovaginal fistulas may present with feces, flatus, or mucus per the vagina.
- Fistulous tract on T2-weighted images or inversion recovery MRI appears as a tract of fluid signal intensity surrounded by lower-signal-intensity granulation tissue and fibrosis. Changes in normal structures in the pelvis are evident on MR images: fascial and muscle edema; thickening of the rectum wall, bladder, and vagina; and fatty infiltration of bone marrow. They depend on the radiation dose and the time elapsed since RT. Increased signal intensity on T2W images usually reflects acute or subacute changes and does not persist indefinitely. Increased signal intensity should not be confused with tumor recurrence.

V. Panebianco, J.J. Fütterer, *MDCT and MRI in Genitourinary Imaging*,   47
A-Z Notes in Radiological Practice and Reporting,
DOI 10.1007/978-88-470-5705-0_6, © Springer-Verlag Italia 2015

Fournier Gangrene

- Fournier gangrene is a necrotizing fasciitis of the perineum. It's a urologic emergency with a potentially high mortality rate; it is typically seen in diabetic men aged about 50–70.
- Clinical presentation: Perineal/scrotal pain, swelling, redness, crepitus from soft tissue gas, systemically unwell, fever, and leukocytosis.
- Although the diagnosis of Fournier gangrene is often made clinically, radiologic imaging—particularly CT—can help confirm the diagnosis and to determine disease extent. The CT features of Fournier gangrene include soft tissue thickening and inflammation, demonstrating the asymmetric fascial thickening; any coexisting fluid collection or abscess; fat stranding around the involved structures; and subcutaneous emphysema secondary to gas-forming bacteria.

Fallopian Tube Cancer

- Primary fallopian tube carcinoma is a rare malignancy that originates from the fallopian tube. They account from 1 to 2 % of all gynecological cancers. It typically presents in postmenopausal women aged 60–79. However, fallopian tube carcinoma has been reported in young girls aged 17–19. The most common histological type of PFTC is papillary serous carcinoma, which is histologically identical to serous ovarian adenocarcinoma.

Most patients are asymptomatic and often insidious; when symptomatic, the most common nonspecific symptoms include Latzko's triad consisting of lower abdominal pain, serosanguineous vaginal discharge, and an adnexal mass (reported in 15 % of cases).

- Most of the tumors originate from the ampulla with an 0endoluminal growth that leads to hydrosalpinx. Fallopian tube cancer can be bilateral in 20 % of the cases. The most common histological types are serous and endometrioid carcinoma, with a pattern of growth nodular, papillary, infiltrative, or mass forming.
- The lesion can have the appearance of a small, solid, lobulated mass on CT scan or on MRI. Advanced tumors are difficult to differentiate from ovarian tumors on imaging. The presence of a hydrosalpinx can be a useful feature.
- On CT scan, the lesion has an attenuation equal to that of other soft tissue masses and enhances less than the myometrium.
- On T1 images, the solid tumor portion is usually hypointense; if there is an associated simple hemorrhagic fluid containing hydrosalpinx, this may be of high signal. On T2 images, the solid tumor component is often homogeneously hyperintense. After somministration of gadolinium contrast, T1 images of the solid portion often demonstrate enhancement. MRI seems to be better than CT scan or ultrasound in detecting tumor infiltration of the bladder, vagina, pelvic sidewalls, pelvic fat, and rectum.
- Data from the literature indicate that patients with PFTC have a higher rate of retroperitoneal and distant metastases. Metastases to the para-aortic lymph nodes have been documented in 33 % of the patients with all stages of disease.

Suggested Reading

Callahan TL, Caughey AB. 2008. Blueprints Obstetrics and Gynecology. Lippincott Williams & Wilkins. ISBN:078178249X.

Haaga JR, Lanzieri CF and Gilkeson RC. 2003. CT and MR imaging of the whole body. Fourth Edition, Mosby.

Eurorad teaching files: Case 7075.

Pectasides D, Pectasides E and Economopoulos T. 2006. Fallopian Tube
    Carcinoma: A Review. Oncologist.

Levenson RB, Singh AK and Novelline RA. 2008. Fournier Gangrene: Role
    of Imaging.

Kim MY, Rha SE, Oh SN et al. 2009. MR Imaging findings of hydrosal-
    pinx: a comprehensive review. Radiographics. 29 (2): 495–507.

G

Germ Cell Tumor, Ovarian

- Ovarian germ cell neoplasms (OGCNs) may be benign or malignant. These neoplasms comprise approximately 20–25 % of ovarian neoplasms overall and arise primarily in young women aged between 10 and 30.
- Germ cell tumors are a histologically heterogeneous group of tumors. The main categories of ovarian germ cell tumor are teratomas (the most common benign OGCNs), immature teratomas, dysgerminomas, endodermal sinus or yolk sac tumors, and mixed germ cell tumors. These conditions are bilateral in 10–12 % of cases, while the majority of other histologies present as unilateral ovarian masses. OGCNs often produce hormones, particularly the beta subunit of human chorionic gonadotropin (hCG), and grow rapidly.
- Patients typically present with one or more symptoms: abdominal enlargement (from the mass itself, ascites, or both; in 87 % of patients), abdominal pain (from rupture, hemorrhage, or torsion; in 85 % of patients), precocious puberty, abdominal distention, fever, abnormal vaginal bleeding (presumably from hCG production), and symptoms of pregnancy (from hCG production).

V. Panebianco, J.J. Fütterer, *MDCT and MRI in Genitourinary Imaging*, 51
A-Z Notes in Radiological Practice and Reporting,
DOI 10.1007/978-88-470-5705-0_7, © Springer-Verlag Italia 2015

- In virtually all cases, surgery is required for definitive histological diagnosis, treatment, and staging (if malignant) of OGCNs.
- *CT* has high sensitivity in the diagnosis of *cystic teratomas*. Typically, CT images demonstrate fat, fat–fluid level, and calcifications. The presence of most of the above tissues is diagnostic of ovarian cystic teratomas in 98 % of cases. Malignant transformation should be suspected if the size exceeds 10 cm or if a mass with irregular borders is seen. When ruptured, the characteristic hypoattenuating fatty fluid can be found typically below the right hemidiaphragm.

  - *Immature teratoma*: On CT images, punctate foci of fat and scattered calcifications are indicative of teratoma. The cystic components contain serous fluid or more rarely sebaceous or adipose material. The imaging appearance is typically of a large, heterogeneous mass with fatty elements, coarse irregular calcifications, and numerous cysts of variable sizes. However, the spectrum of appearances ranges from a predominantly cystic to a predominantly solid mass. Hemorrhage may be present.
  - *Ovarian dysgerminoma*: At imaging, it appears predominantly as a solid, multilocular, and well-defined lesion. CT is able to visualize punctate calcifications and areas of attenuation due to necrosis or hemorrhage. After contrast medium administration, the malignancy shows marked enhancement, especially in the fibrovascular enhancing septa, calcification may be present in a speckled pattern.
  - *Ovarian yolk sac tumor*: The tumor typically appears as a large mass that contains both solid and cystic components. It may extend into the abdomen; bilaterality is rare.
  - *Ovarian choriocarcinoma*: On imaging, choriocarcinomas appear as highly vascular solid tumors with cystic, hemorrhagic, and necrotic areas.

- *MRI* evaluation of *cystic teratomas* usually tends to be reserved for difficult cases but is exquisitely sensitive to fat components. On MR, the lesion appears oval with well-defined margins and elevated signal in T1-weighted sequences and low signal in fat-saturated T1-weighted images. In T2-weighted images, the signal may be variable, although it tends to be similar to that of subcutaneous adipose tissue. The calcifications may not be visible on MR images or may be identifiable as areas of low signal intensity. Enhancement is also able to identify solid invasive components and as such can be used to accurately locally stage malignant variants. Extension through the tumor capsule may be present.

  - *Immature teratoma*: On MR, the small foci of fat have elevated signal intensity in T1-weighted images which fall in fat-suppressed sequences. The solid component has a wide variety of signal intensities at T2-weighted MR imaging. It may metastasize to the peritoneum, liver, or lung.
  - *Ovarian dysgerminoma*: On MR, dysgerminoma appears with low signal intensity relative to the muscle on T1-weighted images and isointense on T2 where the fibro-vascular septa appear hypointense to isointense and the areas of necrosis hyperintense. Similar to CT, the septations may show marked contrast enhancement.
  - *Ovarian yolk sac tumor*: Their main feature on MRI is prominent signal voids. The bright dot sign is an enhancing foci in the wall or solid components. Areas of hemorrhage are common. Areas of hemorrhage have high signal intensity on T1-weighted MR images.
  - *Ovarian choriocarcinoma*: Abnormal large signal voids that represent vascular structures and small cystic cavities are seen in solid components at T2-weighted MR imaging, and high-signal-intensity foci, a result of hemorrhage, may be seen in solid portions at T1-weighted MR imaging.

Glomerulonephritis

- Glomerulonephritis is a term used to refer to several renal diseases. Many of the diseases are characterized by inflammation either of the glomeruli or small blood vessels in the kidneys, hence the name; but not all diseases necessarily have an inflammatory component.
- Although there are many causes of glomerular disease, most patients present with one of two patterns, nephrotic or nephritic, that are based upon the urine sediment and the degree of proteinuria.
- The role of CT in renal parenchymal disease is limited but may be useful in selected cases. Non-contrast CT is useful in detecting renal parenchymal calcifications. For patients with renal parenchymal disease, contrast enhancement should be avoided if possible. Contrast-enhanced CT scan may provide useful information regarding the pattern of contrast enhancement and excretion in patients with impaired renal function. Globally absent nephrogram is due to pedicle trauma in most cases, and segmental absence may be due to focal infarction, pyelonephritis, or acute renal failure secondary to renal vasoconstriction.
- Recent advances in MR imaging such as breath-holding rapid imaging technique and renal functional MR imaging such as dynamic contrast-enhanced study, diffusion-weighted (DW) study, and blood oxygen level-dependent (BOLD) study extended the role of MR imaging in the evaluation of renal parenchymal diseases. Gadolinium-based contrast media are used routinely for MR imaging of the kidney. Most normal kidneys show a distinct contrast between the renal cortex and medulla on T1-weighted images, whereas the signal intensities of the renal cortex and medulla are similar on T2-weighted images. Obliteration of the corticomedullary contrast on T1-weighted spin-echo image is regarded as a

sensitive but nonspecific finding of the renal parenchymal disease. The parenchymal enhancement pattern is more clearly demonstrated on gradient-echo imaging than on T1-weighted spin-echo imaging. DW and BOLD MR imaging may yield information on kidney function. Both techniques provide highly reproducible results in patients with good renal function and hold promise for noninvasive monitoring.

Gonadoblastoma

- Gonadoblastoma is a rare benign tumor that has the potential for malignant transformation and affects a subset of patients with an intersex disorder or disorder of sex development (DSD). Most of these tumors are identified within the first two decades of life.
- Gonadoblastoma does not demonstrate invasive behavior; however, 50 % of the specimens demonstrate evidence of local overgrowth by the germinal component, and approximately 10 % of these germinomas/seminomas arising within this context have demonstrated metastases.
- Imaging studies are useful in diagnosing features of intersexuality in newborns but have a limited role in the diagnosis of gonadoblastoma. All of these studies help to identify patients at risk of developing gonadoblastoma in addition to characterizing the specific intersex disorder. In patients that present later in life, localization studies such as ultrasonography, CT scanning, and MRI may be useful. The tumor appearance is similar to that of dysgerminoma, except that in dysgerminoma arising from gonadoblastoma, there are often calcifications (rarely found in pure dysgerminomas).

Suggested Reading

Zalei Y, Piura B, Elchalal U, et al. 1996. Diagnosis and management of malignant germ cell ovarian tumors in young females. Int J Gynaecol Obstet; 55:1.

Tewari K, Cappuccini F, Disaia PJ, et al. 2000. Malignant germ cell tumors of the ovary. Obstet Gynecol; 95:128.

Yamaoka T, Togashi K, Koyama T et-al. 2000. Yolk sac tumor of the ovary: radiologic-pathologic correlation in four cases. J Comput Assist Tomogr; 24: 605–9.

H

Hemangioma

- Hemangioma is a rare mesenchymal benign tumor of the *bladder*, which accounts for 0.6 % of all bladder tumors. The most common symptom is gross, painless hematuria.
- CT scans have been reported to detect diffuse thickening of the bladder wall with multiple loci of calcification or extravesical extension. CT scans were also useful in revealing a hypervascular mass of the bladder in the present case.
- MR imaging has been reported to be valuable in the diagnosis of soft tissue hemangiomas. Hemangiomas demonstrate relatively low signal intensity on T1-weighted images and an intense signal on T2-weighted images. These MR images reflect the content of the lesions, that is, stagnant or slowly flowing blood. MR imaging is useful in defining the extent, size, and location of the tumor in three dimensions. MR imaging has been reported to be superior to CT and US in demonstrating the extent of hemangioma.

V. Panebianco, J.J. Fütterer, *MDCT and MRI in Genitourinary Imaging*, 57
A-Z Notes in Radiological Practice and Reporting,
DOI 10.1007/978-88-470-5705-0_8, © Springer-Verlag Italia 2015

Hemangiopericytoma

- Hemangiopericytoma (HPC) is one of the rarest renal tumors. HPC is an unusual perivascular tumor, classified as a soft tissue vascular tumor featuring the uncontrolled proliferation of pericytes, which are cells spiralling around capillaries.
- No characteristic signs of renal HPC have been described on ultrasonography, CT, or MRI that might aid in the differential diagnosis. These studies usually depict a large mass, which may grow insidiously to a diameter of 25 cm, but with no pathognomonic features. CT may show a large heterogeneous mass, with calcifications and areas of necrosis. These tumors may have a characteristic pattern in the early arterial phase of angiography, with displacement of the main arteries, presence of large vessels encircling the tumor, and a well-demarcated tumor stain.

Hemorrhage, Renal

- The most common cause of renal hemorrhage is trauma, either blunt or penetrating. Extracorporeal shock wave lithotripsy for nephrolithiasis is not infrequently associated with parenchymal and perinephric hemorrhage. Spontaneous renal hemorrhage may be caused by anticoagulation, blood dyscrasias, renal infarction, polyarteritis nodosa, renal aneurysms and arteriovenous malformations, renal cell carcinoma (RCC), acute myeloid leukemia, renal abscess, renal vein thrombosis, and rupture of hemorrhagic solitary cysts or of hemorrhagic cysts in renal cystic disease. Some cases are idiopathic. RCC is probably the most common cause of spontaneous subcapsular and perinephric hemorrhage.
- CT is the most valuable examination in the evaluation of patients with suspected acute renal hemorrhage because it accurately diagnoses the presence and location of such hemorrhage and

often shows the underlying cause. Renal hemorrhage may be suburothelial, intraparenchymal, subcapsular, perinephric, or pararenal in location or may involve the renal sinus. Recent renal hemorrhage is characterized by high-attenuation blood, which is best shown by unenhanced CT scans. Postcontrast scans should also be obtained to facilitate identification of disorders such as small neoplasms causing spontaneous renal hemorrhage. Suburothelial hemorrhage is characterized on CT by thickening of the wall of the renal pelvis and upper ureter by blood that has a high-attenuation value on unenhanced scans. Spontaneous hemorrhage into the renal sinus is characterized by a high-density blood collection in the renal sinus with displacement of the renal pelvis. On an unenhanced CT scan, a recent subcapsular hematoma is characterized by a mass with a higher attenuation value than that of adjacent renal parenchyma. Pressure on the underlying renal parenchyma characteristically causes flattening of the kidney, elevation of the renal capsule, and medial displacement of the collecting system. However, although subcapsular hematomas are confined to the kidney by the renal capsule, perinephric hematomas often extend caudally below the kidney into the cone of renal fascia.

Hernia, Inguinal

- An hernia is defined as a protrusion or projection of an organ or a part of an organ through the body wall that normally contains it. Collectively, inguinal and femoral hernias are known as groin hernias.
- Inguinal hernia is more common than femoral hernia and other abdominal wall hernias (e.g., umbilical, epigastric), but femoral hernias present with complications more often. Groin hernias are the third leading cause of ambulatory care visits for gastrointestinal complaints.

- Hernias are more common in men compared with women and in whites compared with nonwhites. Indirect inguinal hernias are the most common type of hernia in males and females.
- Groin hernias can broadly be classified by etiology (congenital versus acquired) and anatomical location.
- In the majority of cases, a diagnosis of inguinal or femoral hernia can be made based upon history and physical examination, without the need for further studies. When the diagnosis is not apparent, imaging can help to identify occult hernia, differentiate inguinal from femoral hernia, and distinguish hernia from other clinical entities. Imaging is also important for evaluating patients for hernia complications.
- CT of the groin region can help differentiate femoral from inguinal hernias. Sufficiently thin slices using multidetector CT may allow localization of the hernia sac. If the hernia sac extends medial to the pubic tubercle on CT, a diagnosis of inguinal hernia can be made with certainty, but an hernia sac located lateral to the pubic tubercle associated with venous compression suggests a diagnosis of femoral hernia.
- Magnetic resonance imaging (MRI) appears to differentiate inguinal from femoral hernia with a sensitivity and specificity of more than 95 %, which is superior to computed tomography. However, cost and lack of uniform availability limit the practicality of MRI.

Horseshoe Kidney

- Horseshoe kidney is the most common fusion anomaly, which occurs with fusion of one pole of each kidney.
- The majority of patients with horseshoe kidneys are asymptomatic. In these patients, the horseshoe kidney is diagnosed serendipitously. However, some patients present with pain and/or hematuria due to obstruction or infection.

Hydronephrosis is reported to occur in approximately 80 % of children with horseshoe kidneys. Renal calculi are reported to occur in 20 % of cases. Patients with a horseshoe kidney are at increased risk for infection. One-third to one-half of patients with horseshoe kidneys will have another congenital anomaly.

- CT and MR are able to fully visualize the malformed urinary tract: in more than 90 % of cases, fusion occurs at the lower poles; as a result, two separate excretory renal units and ureters are maintained. The isthmus (fused portion) may lie over the midline (symmetric horseshoe kidney) or lateral to the midline (asymmetric horseshoe kidney). Depending on the degree of fusion, the isthmus can be composed of renal parenchyma or a fibrous band.

Hydrocele

- A hydrocele is a collection of peritoneal fluid between the parietal and visceral layers of the tunica vaginalis, the investing layer that directly surrounds the testis and spermatic cord.
- Hydroceles are believed to arise from an imbalance of secretion and reabsorption of fluid from the tunica vaginalis. Hydroceles range in size from small, soft collections that still allow palpation of the scrotal contents to massive, tense collections of several liters that make examination impossible.
- Symptoms of pain and disability generally increase with the size of the mass. Inflammatory conditions of the scrotal contents (epididymitis, torsion, appendiceal torsion) can produce an acute reactive hydrocele, which often resolves with treatment of the underlying condition. Hydroceles discovered in infancy are usually "communicating," since they are associated with a patent processus vaginalis, which allows flow of peritoneal fluid into the scrotal sac. They usually

disappear in recumbent position and are often associated with herniation of abdominal contents (indirect hernia) through the processus vaginalis. Surgical repair is advised in these cases.

- On MRI, hydroceles are characterized by a low signal in T1-weighted images and a high signal in T2-weighted images. This reflects the content of the hydrocele, that is, simple fluid.

Hydronephrosis

- Hydronephrosis, a direct consequence of urinary tract obstruction (UTO), is a relatively common problem. The obstruction to urinary flow may be acute or chronic, partial or complete, and unilateral or bilateral and may occur at any site in the urinary tract.
- The major causes of UTO vary with the age of the patient. Anatomic abnormalities (including urethral valves or stricture and stenosis at the ureterovesical or ureteropelvic junction) account for the majority of cases in children. In comparison, calculi are most common in young adults, while prostatic hypertrophy or carcinoma, retroperitoneal or pelvic neoplasms, and calculi are the primary causes in older patients.
- The clinical manifestations of UTO vary with the site, degree, and rapidity of onset of the obstruction. Pain is frequently present, due to distention of the bladder, collecting system, or renal capsule; patients with complete or severe partial bilateral obstruction also may develop acute or chronic renal failure; urinary findings are generally nondiagnostic with the only possible exception of anuria; hypertension is occasionally induced by UTO.

- Early diagnosis of UTO is important, since most cases can be corrected and a delay in therapy can lead to irreversible renal injury.
- CT scanning should be performed if the ultrasound results are equivocal or the kidneys cannot be well visualized or if the cause of the obstruction cannot be identified. The combination of a plain film of the abdomen (including tomographic cuts to detect radiopaque calculi), ultrasonography, and, if necessary, CT scanning will be adequate for diagnostic purposes in over 90 % of cases.
- Diffusion-weighted MR imaging may allow noninvasive detection of changes in renal perfusion and diffusion that occur during acute ureteral obstruction. The advantage of this method is that it does not require the use of contrast agents.

Suggested Reading

1. Khadra MH, Pickard RS, Charlton M, et al. 2000. A prospective analysis of 1,930 patients with hematuria to evaluate current diagnostic practice. J Urol; 163:524.
2. Amano T, Kunimi K, Hisazumi H et al. 1993. Magnetic Resonance Imaging of Bladder Hemangioma Abdom Imaging; 18:97–99.
3. Cocheteux B, Mounier-Vehier C, Gaxotte V et al. 2001. Rare variations in renal anatomy and blood supply: CT appearances and embryological background. A pictorial essay. Eur Radial; 11: 779–786.
4. Argyropoulos A, Liakatas I, Lykourinas M. 2005. Renal haemangiopericytoma: the characteristics of a rare tumour BJU International; 95:943–947.

I

Incontinence

- Urinary incontinence is more common in women, and it is related to pelvic organ prolapse and other pelvic floor abnormalities. It is commonly divided into three subtypes: stress, urge, and mixed.
- MRI is acquiring a primary role in evaluating stress incontinence. Sagittal T2-weighted MRI identifies a cystocele as a posteriorly bulging bladder into the vagina. Ultrafast, large-field-of-view, T2-weighted sequences such as single-shot fast spin echo (SSFSE, GE Healthcare scanners) or half-Fourier acquisition turbo spin echo (HASTE, Siemens Medical Solutions scanners) are usually performed for a detailed dynamic pelvic floor visualization during straining; alternatively, true fast imaging in steady-state precession may be performed. Stress incontinence is associated with a greater vesicourethral angle and a larger retropubic space than found in continent women.
- In men, incontinence is generally due to sphincter dysfunction, such as scarring or decreased contractions, after prostatectomy; these findings are evaluated with endourethral US.

V. Panebianco, J.J. Fütterer, *MDCT and MRI in Genitourinary Imaging*, 65
A-Z Notes in Radiological Practice and Reporting,
DOI 10.1007/978-88-470-5705-0_9, © Springer-Verlag Italia 2015

Infarction, Bladder

- Bladder overdistention can lead to ischemia and eventually to gangrene. It can also be secondary to a strangulated bladder in an inguinal hernia, generally in association with herniation of bowel loops and fat tissue.
- CT: Bladder overdistention is often an incidental finding, especially in unconscious patients. Dome of bladder may extend above the level of the umbilicus.

Infarction, Renal

- It is more often secondary to sudden occlusion of renal artery supply, but it can also be secondary to vessel compression by extrinsic tumors, artery thrombosis, emboli, vasculitides, and venous occlusions. One result of renal ischemia is renovascular hypertension, but in some patients, ischemia manifests primarily as renal failure (also called *ischemic nephropathy*).
- CT: Contrast-enhanced CT is the best imaging tool. A focal infarction appears as a wedge-shaped region of decreased or absent contrast enhancement with sharply defined margins, most often extending to the capsule (Fig. 3a, b). Postcontrast CT of a total infarct shows a hypodense, nonfunctioning kidney; prominent capsular collaterals, called the *cortical rim sign*, often lead to surrounding vascular enhancement. If the infarction is chronic, it shows a small kidney with smooth or irregular contour, with no cortical rim sign.
- MRI: A focal infarction appears as a wedge-shaped region with low signal intensity both on T1 and T2; after contrast administration, it shows as a sharply demarcated, nonenhanced tissue. The cortical rim sign can be appreciated; however, this is only seen in around 50 % of the cases.

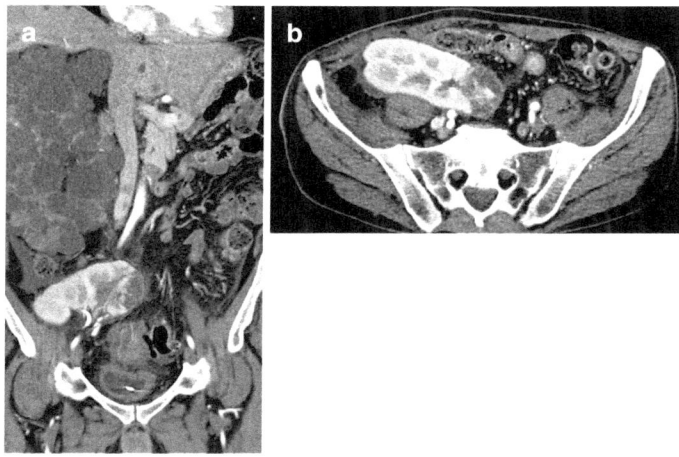

Fig. 3 (**a**, **b**) Coronal and axial CT images showing a wedge-shaped region of decreased contrast enhancement with sharply defined margins, extending to the capsule on the medial aspect of a transplanted pelvic kidney, consistent with renal infarction

Infarction, Testis

- It may result from torsion or trauma, but testicular infarction, although rare, has been also reported as a potential serious complication of a severe or unresolving epididymitis.
- US is the imaging modality of choice; it shows a focal hypoechoic and avascular area on color Doppler.

Suggested Reading

1. Blaivas M, Sierzenski P and Lambert M. 2001. Emergency evaluation of patients presenting with acute scrotum using bedside ultrasonography. Acad Emerg Med.; 8:90–3.

2. Mazeh H, et al. 2008. Laparoscopic inguinal hernia repair on a general surgery ward: 5 years experience. J Laparoendosc Adv Surg Tech A. 18(3):373–6.
3. Yan ML, and Fielding JR. 2008. MRI of Pelvic Floor Dysfunction: *Review*. AJR Volume 191, Number 6.
4. Sue SR, Pelucio M and Gibbs M. 1998. Testicular infarction in a patient with epididymitis. Acad Emerg Med. 5: 1128–30.

J

Juxtaglomerular Cell Tumor

- It is a very rare benign renin-secreting tumor of the kidney, and it can be an unusual cause of secondary hypertension. This tumor is typically found in young adults (with a peak incidence in the second and third decades), and it is reported in children only occasionally. The patients usually present with hypertension, hyperaldosteronism, and hypokalemia, secondary to tumor renin secretion. An occasional incidentally discovered reninoma is nonfunctioning.
- CT: Most juxtaglomerular cell tumors are visible on CT imaging. On unenhanced CT, it usually appears as a unilateral well-circumscribed hypoattenuating cortical mass; most lesions are smaller than 2–3 cm in diameter. At multiphase CT, the tumors are not enhanced in the arterial phase despite the profuse vascularity, possibly because of renin-induced vasoconstriction. The tumors show moderate enhancement during the delayed phase.
- MRI is a powerful diagnostic procedure. At MRI, JCT may appear as a cortical renal mass of variable signal intensity; it appears as an iso-signal intensity cortical lesion on

V. Panebianco, J.J. Fütterer, *MDCT and MRI in Genitourinary Imaging*, 69
A-Z Notes in Radiological Practice and Reporting,
DOI 10.1007/978-88-470-5705-0_10, © Springer-Verlag Italia 2015

T1-weighted images and a high-signal-intensity lesion on T2-weighted images. It shows a delayed peripheral enhancement on dynamic contrast-enhanced MRI.

Suggested Reading

1. Sakata R, Shimoyamada H, Yanagisawa M, et al. 2013. Nonfunctioning juxtaglomerular cell tumor. Case Rep Pathol. 2013.
2. Shera AH, Baba AA, Bakshi IH, et al. 2011. Recurrent malignant juxtaglomerular cell tumor: A rare cause of malignant hypertension in a child. J Indian Assoc Pediatr Surg. 16(4): 152–154.
3. Kuroda N, Gotoda H, Ohe C, et al. 2011. Review of juxtaglomerular cell tumor with focus on pathobiological aspect. Diagnostic Pathology.
4. Katabathina VS, Vikram R, Nagar AM, Tamboli P, Menias CO, Prasad SR. Mesenchymal neoplasms of the kidney in adults: imaging spectrum with radiologic-pathologic correlation. Radiographics. 2010 Oct;30(6):1525–40.

K

Kidney, Ureter, Bladder Plain Film

- KUB can be diagnostic of urinary stones, since 90 % are radiopaque. It is necessary for the follow-up of stone passage or for lithotripsy planning and survey. It can miss small stones, radiolucent urate stones, or stones overlying bone.
- Sometimes phleboliths, vascular calcifications, calcified lymph nodes, appendicoliths, granulomas, various calcified masses, and even bowel contents can be confused with urinary tract stones. KUB taken prior to conventional contrast studies is necessary for their detection.

Kidney Fusion Anomalies

- Congenital variations and malformations of the kidneys that have embryological reasons and lead to fusion of two kidneys, usually at the lower pole, that then form a joined organ in atypical position and rotation, and thus may be accompanied by urinary tract diversion or obstruction. Typical examples are the cross fused or horseshoe kidney.

V. Panebianco, J.J. Fütterer, *MDCT and MRI in Genitourinary Imaging*, 71
A-Z Notes in Radiological Practice and Reporting,
DOI 10.1007/978-88-470-5705-0_11, © Springer-Verlag Italia 2015

Suggested Reading

1. Albert L. Baert – 2007. Encyclopedia of imaging Vol. 2.

L

Leiomyomatous Tumors, Uterus

- Uterine leiomyoma (uterine fibroid) is a benign tumor of myometrial (smooth muscle) origin; it is the most common solid benign uterine neoplasm. Its prevalence increases with age and it is more common in black than in white women. It can be solitary or multiple, with different locations within the uterus: intramural (most common), subserosal, and submucosal, some even being pedunculated.
- CT: CT imaging is not the investigation of choice for the characterization of pelvic masses. Uterine fibroids are often an incidental finding on CT scans performed for other reasons. The typical finding is an enlarged and irregular uterus or a mass in continuity with the uterus. 4 % of fibroids contain calcifications. Most myomas enhance with contrast similar to normal myometrium.
- MRI: MRI is the preferred method for accurately characterizing and localizing pelvic masses. Nondegenerated leiomyomas appear isointense to hypointense on T1-weighted images and hypointense on T2-weighted images. The routine use of

V. Panebianco, J.J. Fütterer, *MDCT and MRI in Genitourinary Imaging*,   73
A-Z Notes in Radiological Practice and Reporting,
DOI 10.1007/978-88-470-5705-0_12, © Springer-Verlag Italia 2015

gadolinium has been shown not to contribute to either fibroid detection or characterization.

Leiomyomatosis

- Diffuse leyomiomatosis is a rare condition that consists of diffuse involvement of the myometrium by innumerable small fibroids, which results in symmetrical enlargement of the uterus.
- Although it is a completely benign condition, there may be dissemination through the peritoneal cavity or occasionally metastases to distant organs.

Leiomyosarcoma, Uterus

- It is a rare malignant tumor, composed entirely of smooth muscle. It accounts for one-third of uterine sarcomas. It may arise in a previously existing benign leiomyoma (sarcomatous transformation) or independently from the smooth muscle cells of the myometrium. Rapid growth and extensive metastasis are frequently encountered with leiomyosarcomas.
- CT: Leiomyosarcoma appear as either a massive uterine enlargement with multiple sarcomatous nodules and irregular central zones of low attenuation, suggesting extensive necrosis and hemorrhage or extensive invasion. Calcifications may be present.
- MRI: Although it has been suggested that an irregular margin of a uterine leiomyoma at MR imaging and a heterogeneous MRI signal are suggestive of sarcomatous transformation, the specificity of these findings has not been established yet. MR imaging findings are variable and include a lobulated mass of high signal intensity on T2-weighted images, a sharply marginated mass of low signal intensity that closely resembles a leiomyoma, or a mass with focally infiltrative margins.

Lipoleiomyomas

- Lipoleiomyomas are rare fat-containing fibroids.
- MRI: they typically show high signal intensity on T1 and low signal intensity on T2-weighted images. Fat-suppression techniques are helpful to confirm the presence of fat.

Lymphangiomyomatosis, Renal

- It consists in a lymphatic developmental malformation, resulting in cystic mass perirenal, peripelvic, and intrarenal regions. The lesions may be unilateral or bilateral and diffuse or focal. It is characterized by cortical dilated endothelial-lined spaces, without glomerular or tubular abnormalities.
- CT: The lesion appears as a subcapsular hypodense mass with fluid density; it has the appearance of a uni- or multi-locular cystic lesion with or without associated peripheral or septal enhancement.
- MRI: Variable signal intensity on T1-weighted images, but usually low signal; high signal intensity on T1-weighted images is seen when the cyst contains proteinaceous material. The cysts have in general high signal intensity on T2-weighted images.

Lymphocele

- It consists in an accumulation of lymph in a cystic structure, with a history of lymph node dissection. A perirenal lympho-cele refers to an abnormal encapsulated collection of lymph within the pelvis; it can potentially occur after renal transplant.
- CT: round, hypoattenuating collection, with water density. It may be bilateral.

Lymphoma/Leukemia, Renal

• Primary renal lymphoma is rare; the kidney is commonly involved by metastatic lymphoma or by direct invasion. Involvement with non-Hodgkin's lymphoma is considerably more common than Hodgkin's lymphoma.
• CT: Renal lymphoma has a wide variety of CT appearances. Typical findings include multiple renal masses, solitary masses, invasion from contiguous retroperitoneal lymphoma, perirenal disease, and diffuse renal infiltration, usually bilateral. Masses are usually homogenous and poorly enhancing.
• MRI: On T1- and T2-weighted images, lymphoma is isointense or slightly hypointense to renal parenchyma; postcontrast it shows minimal heterogeneous enhancement.

Suggested Reading

Rha SE, Byun JY, Jung SE et-al. 2003. CT and MRI of uterine sarcomas and their mimickers. AJR Am J Roentgenol.

Markić D, Valencić M, Maricić A et-al. 2011. Lymphocele and renal transplantation. Acta Med Croatica.

Surabhi VR et al. 2008. Neoplastic and non-neoplastic proliferative disorders of the perirenal space: cross-sectional imaging findings. Radiographics 28(4):1005–1017.

Wilde S, Scott-Barrett S. 2009. Radiological appearances of uterine fibroids. Indian J Radiol Imaging. 19 (3): 222–31.

Urban BA, Fishman EK. 2000. Renal lymphoma: CT patterns with emphasis on helical CT. Radiographics. 20 (1): 197–212.

Murase E, Siegelman ES, Outwater EK et-al. 1999. Uterine leiomyomas: histopathologic features, MR imaging findings, differential diagnosis, and treatment. Radiographics.

M

Mesoblastic Nephroma

- Mesoblastic nephroma is the most common renal tumor identified in the neonatal period and the most frequent benign renal tumor in childhood. Solid, homogeneous, usually large tumor that could mimic a Wilms' tumor. Hemorrhage and necrosis develop in the aggressive and malignant variants, although cystic degeneration is not common.
- Adult mesoblastic nephroma differs from the pediatric one, standing as a different disease, could also mimic other tumors such as cystic hamartomas and adrenal tumors.
- The signal intensity characteristics are similar to those of the normal renal parenchyma. The lesion appears isointense to the kidney on T1-weighted images. The signal is lower than that of the surrounding fat and higher than that of the renal medulla. The mass shows increased signal on T2-weighted images. Contrast-enhanced MRIs show no or minimal contrast enhancement in the mass.

Megaureter

- The term megaureter may refer to two conditions: first one, it represents a sequela of uncorrected massive chronic reflux and can also affect the bladder, whereas the second one is a congenital condition (the width exceeds 10 mm).
- The condition is more often detected in children than adults and is more common on the left side.
- US findings show a massive dilation, consisting in an anechoic signal flanked above and below by two hyper/isoechogenic strips which represent the ureter stretched walls.
- CT/MRI well assesses this anomaly. CT without contrast agent shows an enlarged lumen of the ureter.
- CT urography protocol allows to assess a hyperdense signal originating from the lumen itself, caused by the stagnation of contrast agent.
- MRI findings are similar to CT, except that on heavily T2-weighted sequences it could be possible to evaluate lumen swelling thanks to fluid stasis which gives back a strong hyperintense signal, so no contrast could be required.

Metastases to Kidney

- Metastases to the kidneys are common, with multiple foci and bilateral involvement typical.
- Usual metastases to kidney involved melanoma, thyroid carcinoma, liver, colon, lung and breast cancer, and ovarian carcinoma.
- Renal metastases have a CT, US, and MRI appearance similar to that of renal cell carcinoma or lymphoma.
- CT findings reveal that metastases are hypodense and inhomogeneous on unenhanced CT, whereas contrast-enhanced CT reveals most to have inhomogeneous enhancement. Most enhance less than normal renal parenchyma. Metastatic

thyroid carcinomas, on the other hand, tend to be hyperdense and have variable contrast enhancement. Renal vein invasion is rare with metastatic disease.

Multicystic Dysplastic Kidney

- Multicystic dysplastic kidney (MCDK) or multicystic dysplasia is a condition, which occurs during the fetal life, consisting in an anomaly of kidney development. It is a form of renal dysplasia that is secondary to altered metanephric differentiation during embryogenesis. The kidney itself consists of irregular cysts of varying sizes and has no function. This condition could be only unilateral because complete bilateral involvement is incompatible with life. Depending on the extent of involvement, dysplasia is limited to the infundibula, renal pelvis, and proximal ureter, or it involves a kidney to the point that dilated calyces appear as intrarenal cysts. Segmental multicystic dysplasia occurs in a setting of a duplex collecting system.
- A multicystic dysplastic kidney is commonly associated with vesicoureteral reflux in the contralateral kidney and with a posterior location of the urethral valves.
- Ultrasound is the imaging modality of choice.
- MRI with T2 sequences imaging clearly shows the altered structure of the kidney.
- CT is not recommended since almost all exams are performed on pediatric population.

Malacoplakia of Kidney

- Malacoplakia is a rare, inflammatory process related to an abnormal host response to chronic infection (chronic tubulointerstitial nephritis) characterized by round intra and extracellular inclusion bodies (the eponymic Michaelis–Gutmann bodies).

- Malacoplakia most commonly manifests as a mucosal mass involving the bladder or ureter, the most frequent renal finding is obstruction secondary to a lesion in the lower tract. In approximately 15 % of reported cases, the kidney is identified as the primary site of disease.
- CT: The lesions appear with minimal enhancement on the contrast-enhanced CT and stand out against the vascular blush of the normal renal cortex. The classic appearance is an enlarged kidney with multiple hypovascular masses.
- MRI: Low signal intensity on both T1- and T2-weighted images and delayed enhancement of the fibrous stroma is noticed.

Medullary Carcinoma of Kidney

- Renal medullary carcinoma is a rare collecting duct and a highly aggressive neoplasm that almost always develops in teenagers and young adults with sickle cell trait or hemoglobin SC disease.
- At imaging, these tumors appear as ill-defined, infiltrative masses that arise in the renal medulla and invade the renal sinus; occasionally, a necrotic tumor communicates with the collecting system.
- The lesion is hypointense on T2-weighted images. They show heterogeneous contrast enhancement, presumably due to necrosis.
- Venous invasion and nodal metastases are common.

Multilocular Cystic Tumor of Kidney

- Multilocular cystic tumor of kidney is represented by two entities (Multilocular Cystic Nephroma/Cystic Partially

Differentiated Nephroblastoma); the first one occur in adults, whereas the latter in pediatric patients. Their architecture consists of a mixture of epithelial and mesenchymal components. Imaging detects both of these cystic tumors but cannot differentiate between them. Their appearance is similar to other cystic tumors. They occur unilaterally.

- CT reveals multilocular cystic nephromas to be homogeneous, multicystic tumors containing thin septa without a solid component; for some reason a lower pole location predominates. The cystic component does not enhance with contrast.
- MR imaging of a multilocular cystic nephroma reveals a complex solitary renal cystic tumor often protruding into the renal collecting system and containing thin septa, with the cystic component varying from hypo- to hyperintense on T1-weighted images. Any solid component and septa enhance postcontrast in all cases.

Multidetector CT of Kidney

- Multidetector CT allows imaging during specific contrast opacification phases. MDCT urography with a two-phase (unenhanced and combined nephrographic and excretory phase) split-bolus technique and oral hydration is advised. Using a split-bolus technique, both a nephrogenic and excretory phases can be obtained with one scan, although such a protocol tends not to visualize all of the ureters completely.
- Renal opacification can be divided into three phases: first is an early vascular or bolus phase, then a nephrogram phase (consisting of a nephrogram), followed by a pyelogram or equilibrium (delayed) phase. A corticomedullary phase, providing maximum differentiation between renal cortex and medulla, occurs during the early phase. Both neoplasms and normal renal parenchyma enhance significantly more during

the nephrogram phase than during the corticomedullary phase. In general, more tumors <3 cm in diameter are detected on the nephrogram phase than on the corticomedullary phase.

- Corticomedullary phase is useful for detection of such conditions as an aneurysm, arteriovenous malformation, or fistula, and in evaluating tumor vascularity. Renal tumors tend to be detected with greater confidence on delayed images than on early-phase images.
- Three-dimensional CT imaging techniques are useful both in evaluating suspected tumors.

MRI of Kidney

- MRI is used in a setting of contrast allergy or renal failure and for studying some complex masses. It is also useful in evaluating venous thrombosis in a setting of renal carcinoma.
- MRI evaluates renovascular disease, assesses renal function, detects renal tumors, and identifies urinary tract abnormalities, all without radiation exposure.
- Magnetic resonance signal intensity normally decreases in the pyelocaliceal phase due to contrast agent concentration. When searching for small renal tumors, use of a body phased-array coil in combination with fast low-angle shot (FLASH) and fat suppression pre- and postcontrast thin section MR allow imaging in single breathholds. Sagittal and coronal plane images improve evaluation. Both T1- and T2-weighted sequences are useful with contrast-enhanced MRI to evaluate renal blood flow and renal function. During the early phase, a renal cortex signal increase in T1-weighted sequences is matched by a similar signal decrease in T2-weighted sequences; during later phases, however, T2-weighted sequence signal intensity in the medulla decreases markedly. Thus, renal cortical blood flow can be evaluated with either

sequence, but T2-weighted sequences appear more useful in evaluating renal medulla. Presumably increased amounts of contrast in renal tubules account for the medullary decreased signal intensity during later phase T2-weighted sequences. Serial dynamic MR-gradient echo imaging using a low contrast dose can be used to obtain an intensity–time curve, similar to radionuclide renography.

• A relative disadvantage in certain renal applications is its poor sensitivity in detecting calcifications.

Medullary Sponge Kidney

• Medullary sponge kidney (i.e., Lenarduzzi–Cacchi–Ricci disease) is a congenital developmental abnormality characterized by ectasia and cystic dilatation of the intrapyramidal or intrapapillary portions of the renal medullary collecting ducts. Among patients with calcific kidney stones, 12–20 % have medullary sponge kidney.

• In general this disease is asymptomatic. Symptoms which can be observed in patients are hematuria, renal colic, fever, and dysuria.

• Ultrasound: An echogenic appearance of the medullary pyramids is characteristic of medullary sponge kidney.

• CT: CT urography may show a characteristic papillary blush and associated calculi within the dilated collecting ducts.

Suggested Reading

Runge VM. 2013. Current technological advances in magnetic resonance with critical impact for clinical diagnosis and therapy. Invest. Radiol. Dec;48(12):869–77. doi: 10.1097/01.rli.0000434380.71793.d3.

Curry NS, Cochran ST, Bissada NK. 2000. Cystic renal masses: accurate Bosniak classification requires adequate renal CT.AJR; 175:339–342.

Israel GM, Hindman N, Bosniak MA. 2004. Evaluation of cystic renal masses: comparison of CT and MR imaging by using the Bosniak classification system. Radiology;231:365–371.

Tello R, Davison BD, O'Malley M, et al. 2000. Magnetic resonance imaging of renal masses interpreted on CT to be suspicious.AJR;174: 1017–1022.

Rohrschneider WK, Weirich A, Rieden K, et al. 1998. US, CT and MR imaging characteristics of nephroblastomatosis. Pediatr Radiol.

N

Nephrogenic rests. See 'Nephroblastomatosis in Collecting Duct Carcinoma'.

Nephrolithiasis in ureteral calculi. See 'Ureter, Obstruction of'.

Nephroma Mesoblastic, Congenital

- Congenital mesoblastic nephroma, or congenital fetal renal hamartoma, occurs almost exclusively in the first year of life and it is the most common solid renal tumor in the newborn.
- Most patients present with a palpable abdominal mass. Hematuria, hypercalcemia, abdominal pain, and hypertension also occur. It has in general a benign course.
- CT: The tumor appears as a nonenhancing low-attenuation mass within which scattered islands of enhancing residual normal parenchyma.
- MRI: Most common finding on MR imaging are homogeneously low signal intensities on T1-weighted sequences and homogeneously low signal intensities on T2-weighted sequences. Infrequently, areas of necrosis and hemorrhage are seen.

V. Panebianco, J.J. Fütterer, *MDCT and MRI in Genitourinary Imaging*, 85
A-Z Notes in Radiological Practice and Reporting,
DOI 10.1007/978-88-470-5705-0_14, © Springer-Verlag Italia 2015

Nephrostomy, Percutaneous

• Percutaneous nephrostomy is a procedure used mainly in the decompression of the renal collecting system. When the obstructed system becomes infected, and antibiotics are unable to penetrate the kidney and if the purulent material cannot be drained, percutaneous nephrostomy is a resolutive treatment because it allows decompression of the obstructed system, permits specimen collection, and creates a route for antibiotic instillation if needed.

• The indication for CT guidance is limited because most nephrostomies can be performed easily using either fluoroscopic or ultrasound guidance. The indications for which CT guidance may be used are renal transplants, unilateral kidney, high-risk patients, or a kidney with a urinoma associated with hydronephrosis.

• When the nephrostomy is performed under CT guidance, several technical maneuvers are important. Once the collecting system has been penetrated, a small sample of fluid should be aspirated for culture and then a small amount of contrast material should be immediately injected. This permits direct visualization under fluoroscopy when the catheter is being inserted.

Suggested Reading

Bolande RP. 1973. Congenital mesoblastic nephroma of infancy. Perspec Pediatric pathol 1:227–250.

Haaga JR, Lanzieri CF, Gilkeson RC. 2003. CT and MR imaging of the whole body. Fourth Edition, Mosby.

Prasad SR, Humphrey PA, Meninas CO et al. Neoplasms of the Renal Medulla: Radiologic-Pathologic Correlation.

O

Oncocytoma, Renal

- Oncocytoma is the second most common benign renal neo-plasm after angiomyolipoma. It accounts for 3–7 % of solid renal masses. They appear to originate from the cortical part of collecting tubules. These tumors are often detected inci-dentally in asymptomatic individuals; some are multiple, bilateral, or metachronous in a minority of cases. In rare cases, presenting as hundreds of nodules scattered through-out both kidneys.
- CT: they are solid, well-marginated, homogeneous, and often large tumors. Cystic changes and calcifications are rare. They have no specific imaging features (such as MRI), in fact imaging cannot differentiate it from a malignant renal mass, unlike which, hemorrhage and necrosis are not common. Oncocytomas tend to contain a central stellate scar that mim-ics the necrosis seen in a renal cell carcinoma.
- MRI: The MR appearance is variable and nonspecific. They are hypointense on T1-weighted MR images (70 % of the cases) but vary in signal intensity on T2-weighted images (67 % high signal intensity), often with a well-defined

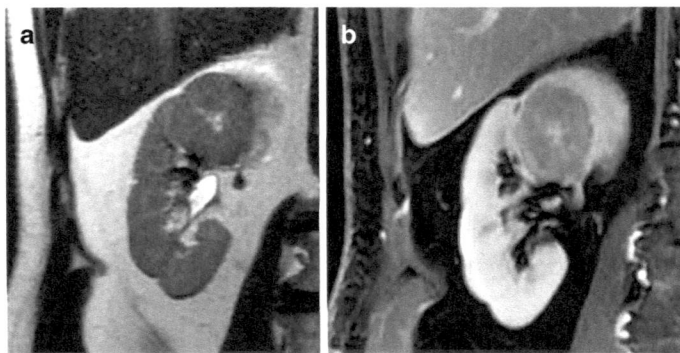

Fig. 4 (**a**, **b**) Oncocytoma in a 40-year-old woman. T2-weighted imaging and delayed contrast-enhanced T1-weighted images, showing a large, round-shaped, well-defined, mass with heterogeneous signal intensity and a central cleft. Oncocytoma was confirmed at histopathology analysis performed after nefrectomy

capsule. The central scar (when present) can be seen as a stellate area of low signal intensity on T1-weighted images and high signal intensity on T2-weighted images; Fig. 4a, b. Postcontrast MR imaging reveals, in a minority of oncocytomas, a "spoke-wheel" enhancement pattern. However, this is a nonspecific sign, because a similar vascular arrangement has been described with renal cell carcinoma.

Orchidopexy

• Orchidopexy is the most succesful surgical treatment of cryptorchidism that is characterized by the failure of descent of one or both testicles in the scrotum. Surgical intervention is aimed at positioning and fixing of one or both testicles. The undescended testes is associated with a greater incidence of neoplasia at this level since the retention leads to degenerative phenomena of the gonad with arrest of spermatogenesis. This procedure should be performed after the twelfth month of life, the period during which the testicle could still end his physiological descent into the scrotum.

- Several complications may occur including testicular retraction, atrophy or infarction, hematoma formation, ilio-inguinal nerve injuring, postoperative torsion, and damage to the vas deference.
- MR imaging can be used in case ultrasound is inconclusive. Anatomical T1- and T2-weighted imaging can be applied for scrotal and pelvic evaluation. The testis is high signal intensity on T2 and intermediate signal intensity on T1.

Orchitis

- Most episodes of orchitis result from extensions of acute epididymitis. In isolated orchitis, a viral infection, such as mumps, should be suspected. Causative agent in adolescent and men younger than 35 years are usually considered as *Chlamydia trachomatis* and *Neisseria gonorrhoeae*. Less common causes of epididymitis and orchitis include Granulomatous conditions such as Tuberculosis, Sarcoidosis, and Brucellosis and chemical epididymitis in reflux of sterile urine, amiodarone therapy, or prostate brachytherapy. In children less than 2 years of age, a predisposing condition is usually identified, such as imperforated anus, ureteral ectopia to seminal vesicles, bladder exstrophy, and posterior urethral valves.
- Complications of epididymo-orchitis are abscess formation, pyocele, infarct, gangrene, infertility, atrophy and chronic pain.
- MRI: In epididymo-orchitis, the testis and epididymis have heterogeneous low signal intensities on T2-weighted images.

The epididymis will be enlarged and hyperenhancing with contrast on T1-weighted studies. The testis may show inhomogeneous enhancement with hypointense bands.

Ovarian, Functional Cyst

• Ovarian cysts are seen in all age groups, and many of them are functional cysts. Functional ovarian cysts include follicular cyst and corpus luteal cyst. Follicular cysts results from a failure of the follicle to rupture and corpus luteum cysts derive from hemorrhage in corpus luteum. Simple cysts have in general a size less than 3 mm. Unilocular cysts have a diameter less than 3 cm. Corpus luteal cysts may be larger and tend to be more symptomatic than follicular cysts. Functional cysts may spontaneously regress over time, usually within two menstrual cycles, and they should be monitored by follow-up US at 6–8 weeks.

MRI: Most ovarian cysts show a thin wall, with a very high signal intensity on T2-weighted images and intermediate to low signal intensity on T1-weighted images because of simple fluid content. Similar imaging characteristics may be seen in benign ovarian cystic tumors. The most helpful feature in distinguishing functional cysts from ovarian neoplasms is the presence of papillary projections and nodular septa in the latter. Larger simple cysts cannot be differentiated from unilocular cystadenoma, but if the cyst is more than 10 cm, a tumorous condition should be considered. The most helpful feature in distinguishing functional cysts from ovarian cystic tumors is the presence of papillary projections and nodular septa in the latter. Corpus luteal cysts have thicker walls than follicular cysts and avid enhancement, due to the thick luteinized cell layer that lines the interior of the cyst. Corpus luteum cysts do not demonstrate the profound T2 shortening that is seen with many endometriomas (T2-shading).

Ovarian Mature Cystic Teratoma

- Teratoma, also known as dermoid cyst, is the most common ovarian neoplasm in woman under 45 years of age. "Mature" means benign, as opposed to the immature, malignant teratoma. Ovarian teratomas derive from germ cells and are classified into three main categories, among which the mature cystic teratoma account for 99 %. Less common types of mature teratomas are the monodermal teratomas, which include the struma ovarii and carcinoid tumors.

- They are slow-growing tumors and most tend to be asymptomatic. Therefore, they are discovered incidentally at imaging. The most commonly associated complication is ovarian torsion; in fact, even though benign, they are often resected; other complications are infection, rupture and, rarely, hemolytic anemia. Malignant transformation can occur but is also rare.

- Up to 90 %, they are unilocular and their diameter is smaller than 10 cm. The cystic component is fluid fat, produced by sebaceous glands in cyst lining, and the presence of fat is diagnostic. Up to 60 % may contain calcifications.

- The inner lining of every mature cystic teratoma contains single or multiple white shiny masses projecting from the wall toward the center of the cysts. When hair, other dermal appendages, bone, and teeth are present, they usually arise from this protuberance known as the Rokitansky protuberance that is a common site of malignant transformation.

- CT images demonstrate fat, fat fluid level, sebum-rich fluid in the cyst cavity, calcification (sometimes tooth) may present or not present in the wall, Rokitansky protuberance (adipose tissue) and tufts of hair. Whenever the size exceeds 10 cm or soft tissue plugs and cauliflower appearance with irregular borders is seen, malignant transformation should be suspected; Fig. 5.

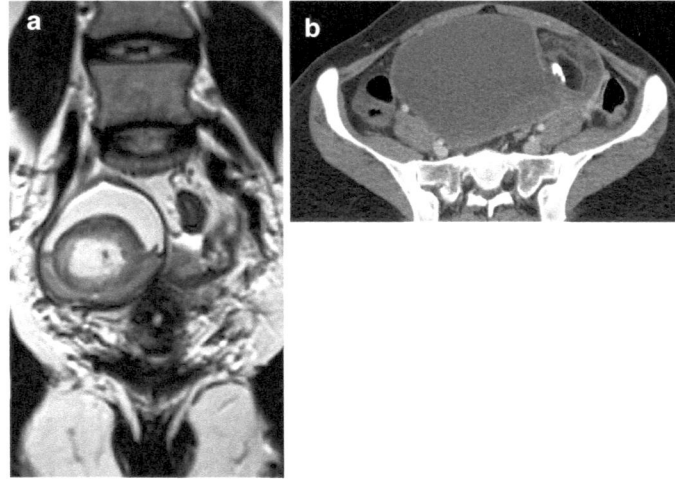

Fig. 5 (**a**) Mature teratoma in a 28-year-old woman. Coronal image of a contrast-enhanced CT scan shows a large cystic tumor with fat and multiple toothlike calcification. (**b**) Axial image of the same CT

MRI: On T1-weighted images, the lipid-laden cyst fluids are hyperintense, while calcifications and fibrosis are hypointense. The fatty regions demonstrate intermediate signal intensity on T2-weighted images; Fig. 6.

Ovarian Cystadenoma

- Ovarian cystadenoma is one of the most common benign ovarian tumors in the reproductive age and this frequency tends to increase with age. There are two different types that differ in pathology, prognosis, and disease: serous and mucinous cystadenoma.
- Both are thin-walled unilocular or multilocular cystic lesions filled with water-like or higher proteinaceous

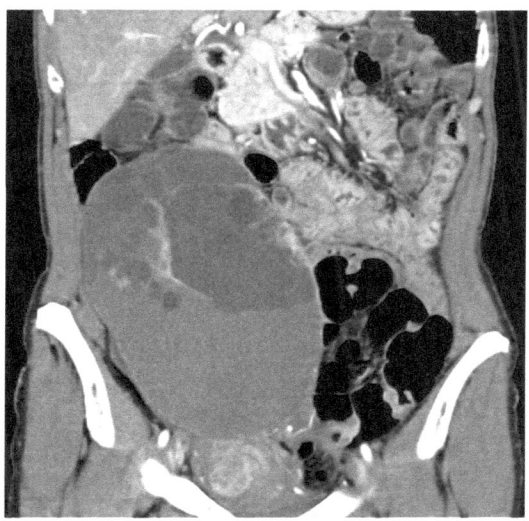

Fig. 6 Mucinous cystadenocarcinoma of right ovarian in a 61-year-old woman. Coronal image of a contrast-enhanced CT scan shows a large multilocular cystic tumor with some thick, enhancing septations and mural nodules. The locules are of different attenuation, consistent with varying protein content

contents. At imaging a serous cystadenoma is most often unilocular and anechoic on ultrasound, and may look like a simple cyst. Mucinous cyst adenomas tend to be filled with sticky gelatinous fluid and are typically multilocular with different contents of the loculi, separated by thin septations and tend to be larger than serous cyst adenomas (mean size of 10 cm). The finding of papillary projections should raise the suspicion of a possible borderline malignancy or a cystadenocarcinoma.

- CT: Cystadenomas are well-circumscribed cystic tumors, with regular and thin (<3 mm) wall and internal septations, that show enhancement.

- MRI: The cystic loculi of serous cystadenomas tend to be low in signal on T1 and high on T2-weighted images because of simple fluid content. The content of the different loculi of mucous cystadenoma varies from watery to proteinaceous to hemorrhagic, in fact have various signal intensities; the sticky gelatinous contents or mucin display intensity higher than water on T2 and lower on T2-weighted images relative to serous fluid.

Ovarian Cystadenofibroma

- Ovarian cystadenofibroma is an uncommon benign epithelial ovarian tumor (1.7 % of ovarian tumors) that displays as cystic tumors with a variable amounts of fibrous stroma.
- The imaging features are nonspecific and vary from purely cystic to a complex cystic tumor with one or more solid components.
- MRI: typically appear as multilocular cystic masses with a solid fibrotic component of low signal intensity on T2-weighted images or cystic wall thickening with a low signal intensity on T2-weighted images without any definite solid component.

Ovarian Carcinoma

- Ovarian cancer is the fifth most common cancer in women and is the leading cause of death from gynecological cancer. The prevalence increases with age, and the peak is reached in the VI-VII decade of life. Tumors arising from the surface epithelium account for 90 % of ovarian cancers and are pathologically designated as serous, mucinous, clear cell, endometrioid, or Brenner (transitional) tumors based on the cell type. Each histologic type is further classified as benign, borderline malignant (tumors of low malignant potential), or malignant, reflecting differences in clinical behavior.

- Onset of symptoms is insidious, in fact 75 % of patients present with advanced (Stage III or IV) disease. Early symptoms are often vague, such as abdominal discomfort, abdominal distension, or bloating, urinary frequency or dyspepsia. It most commonly presents with a pelvic or abdominal mass that may be associated with pain. Often associated with ascites and metastasises to pelvic and periaortic lymph nodes, as well as over the pelvic and abdominal peritoneum.

- Serous cystadenocarcinoma is the most common malignant epithelial tumor cell type, accounting for more than half of epithelial tumors: appears as a multiloculated cystic lesion in content serous or hemorrhagic cloudy or intracystic vegetation.

- CT: Imaging findings that are suggestive of malignant tumors include: a thick, irregular wall, thick septa, papillary projections and a large soft-tissue component with necrosis; see Fig. 6. Ancillary findings of pelvic organ invasion, implants (peritoneal, omental, and mesenteric), ascites, and adenopathy increase diagnostic confidence for malignancy.

- MRI: The cystic loculi tend to be low in signal on T1 and high on T2-weighted images because of simple fluid content. The content of the different loculi varies from watery to proteinaceous to hemorrhagic, in fact have various signal intensities; the solid components have intermediate signal on T1-weighted images and variable on T2-weighted images and post-MR contrast show enhancement.

Ovarian Metastases

- Tumors may metastasize to the ovary by direct extension and through lymphatic, hematogenous, or transperitoneal spreads.

Metastases to the ovaries account for 10 % of ovarian cancer. The most common primary tumors to involve the ovaries are gastrointestinal carcinoma and (in decreasing order of frequency) pancreatic, breast, and uterine carcinomas. The term "Krukenberg tumor" is reserved for metastases to the ovaries in which malignant signet ring cells invade an abundant and hypercellular stroma.

- CT: The tumors are usually solid, but cystic areas are common. Ovarian metastases from colon cancer tend to be unilateral and cystic so can be difficult differentiate them from primary ovarian cancer.
- MRI: The following features are suggestive: bilateral, predominantly solid masses, hypointense solid areas on T2-weighted images, and strong wall enhancement on contrast-enhanced study.

Ovarian Leydig Cell Tumor

- Leydig cell tumors are very rare ovarian neoplasms (less than 0.5 % of all ovarian tumors), belong to the group of steroid cell tumors. They are usually benign and predominantly seen in postmenopausal women. These lesions contain Leydig cells, lutein cells, and adrenocortical cells in various amounts together with a fibrous stroma and are often associated with a virilization syndrome.
- MRI shows small (<3 cm) and unilateral solid masses. The signal on T2 sequence is variable, depending on the extent of fibrous stroma and the lipid components appear as areas of elevated signal on T1- and T2-weighted images. Intense enhancement of the nonfibrotic portions after intravenous administration of gadolinium is usually displayed.

Ovarian Vein Thrombosis

- Ovarian vein thrombosis is an uncommon disorder that may be associated with a variety of inflammatory and malignant conditions. Clinical signs and symptoms are often nonspecific, but prompt recognition and appropriate therapy is essential. Typically, it presents in the setting of postpartum sepsis.
- Untreated, the condition can result in complications such as extension into the inferior vena cava, involvement of the renal veins, or pulmonary embolism.
- CT or MRI may be used to demonstrate the thrombosed veins. Sonography, however, has relatively poor detection rates for OVT, because it may not show the entire length of the vein in most cases secondary to body habitus and overlying bowel gas.
- CT: The thrombosed ovarian vein is visualized as a dilated tubular retroperitoneal structure that contains central low attenuation areas that represent the actual thrombus. Secondary signs associated with OVT are an enlarged uterus that contains fluid and inhomogeneously enhancing parauterine mass believed to be secondary to accompanying pelvic thrombophlebitis.
- MRI can differentiate between acute and subacute thrombus; generally, the ovarian vein clot is subacute (between 1 week and 1 month), with shortened T1 and prolonged T2 relaxation time and, therefore, is hyperintense on both weightings. Time of flight sequence or contrast-enhanced magnetic resonance venography shows thrombus as filling defects.

Suggested Reading

Turgut AT, Bhatt S, Dogra VS. 2008. Acute painful scrotum, Ultrasound clinic; 3: 93–107.

Jung SE, Lee JM, Rha SE et al. 2002. CT and MRI of ovarian tumors with emphasis on the differential diagnosis. Radiographics; 22: 1305–1325

Montoriol PF, Mons A, Da Ines D, et al. 2013. Fibrous tumours of the ovary: Aetiologies and MRI features, Clinical Radiology; 68: 1276–1283

Iyer VR, Lee SI. 2010. MRI, CT, and PET/CT for Ovarian Cancer Detection and Adnexal Lesion Characterization, American Journal of Roentgenology; 194: 311–321

Park SB, Lee JB. 2014. MRI Features of Ovarian Cystic Lesions, Journal of magnetic resonance imaging; doi: 10.1002/jmri.24579

Rosenkrantz AB, Hindman N, Fitzgerald EF, et al. 2010. MRI Features of Renal Oncocytoma and Chromophobe Renal Cell Carcinoma. AJR; 195: 421–427

Virmani V, Kaza R, Sadaf A et al. 2012. Ultrasound, Computed Tomography, and Magnetic Resonance Imaging of Ovarian Vein Thrombosis in Obstetrical and Non obstetrical Patients. Canadian Association of Radiologists Journal; 69: 109–11

Kim W, Rosen MA, Langer JE et al. 2007. US MRI imaging correlation in pathologic conditions of the scrotum. Radiographics; 27: 1239–1253

P

Pelvic Inflammatory Disease

- Pelvic inflammatory disease (PID) is a common condition among women of reproductive age and is usually caused by infection ascending from the endocervix through the uterine cavity.
- Patients usually present with a myriad of nonspecific symptoms, including fever, abdominal or pelvic pain, vaginal discharge, uterine bleeding, dyspareunia, dysuria, adnexal or cervical tenderness, nausea, vomiting, and other vague constitutional symptoms. Laparoscopy, which allows direct visualization of purulent exudates and edema of the pelvic structures, has long been the standard of reference in the diagnosis of PID, but it requires general anesthesia and is an expensive and invasive procedure.
- CT: CT findings are typically subtle early in the course of PID. Mild pelvic edema that results in thickening of the uterosacral ligaments and haziness of the pelvic fat with obscuration of the pelvic fascial planes are seen in the initial phase. Later in the course of PID, the fallopian tubes exhibit an even greater degree of wall thickening and enhancement and fill

V. Panebianco, J.J. Fütterer, *MDCT and MRI in Genitourinary Imaging*, A-Z Notes in Radiological Practice and Reporting, DOI 10.1007/978-88-470-5705-0_16, © Springer-Verlag Italia 2015

with complex fluid, findings that usually indicate pyosalpinx. The abscess manifests as bilateral thick-walled, fluid-filled adnexal masses. The abscess wall and adjacent soft tissue inflammation enhance intensely. Internal gas bubbles, which are unusual, are the most specific sign of an abscess.

- MRI: Tubal enlargement can be easily seen on MR images and is characterized by the tortuous folding of fluid-filled structures on T2-weighted images. Associated findings include thickening of the uterosacral ligaments, infiltration of the presacral fat secondary to edema, hydronephrosis, and indistinct margins of adjacent bowel loops.

Penis Prosthesis

- Penis prosthesis is a treatment option for men with erectile dysfunction. There are two main types of penile implants: semi-rigid and inflatable.
- MRI can clearly demonstrate the position of both semirigid and inflatable prostheses. The saline solution in inflatable devices is well seen with T2-weighted sequences; the silicone in semirigid devices has low signal intensity on T2-weighted images.

Peyronie Disease

- Peyronie disease is a common acquired condition, with a prevalence of around 3 %, associated with penile curvature and a palpable plaque in the tunica albuginea and adjacent corpus cavernosum. The plaque is mostly located unifocally in the penile dorsum with an extension of about 1.5–3 cm causing a typical dorsal deviation. Morphologically, an inflammatory reaction with thickening of the tunica in the beginning, later on a fibrotic, often calcified plaque is typical.

- Plaques from Peyronie disease are usually palpable and are visible at both US and MR imaging in the majority of cases.
- CT is not routinely used and can only show calcification.
- MRI: Plaque formation has been associated with low signal intensity, disruption, localized thickening, and irregularity of the adjacent tunica albuginea with both T1- and T2-weighted sequences. Erection induced by the injection of Prostaglandin E1 stretches the tunica albuginea improving the conditions for plaque detection. The intravenous application of para-magnetic contrast medium leads to an increased local signal intensity (T1-weighted) depending on the degree of tissue perfusion with a focal contrast enhancement around or within the plaques indicating an inflammatory status of the plaque.

Polycystic Kidney Disease

- The Potter classification of renal cystic diseases separates cystic kidneys into four types: (1) infantile polycystic kidney disease; (2) cystic dysplastic kidney disease; (3) adult poly-cystic kidney disease; and (4) partial or intermittent urinary outflow obstruction (obstructive dysplasia).
- *Autosomal Recessive Polycystic Kidney Disease (ARPKD):* also known as Potter type I and infantile polycystic disease, the autosomal-recessive form of polycystic kidney disease manifests early in life. The underlying defect is renal tubular ectasia. The nephrons are normal. Expressivity varies with some patients not surviving beyond the neonatal period. Those with milder renal involvement survive longer and develop hepatobiliary fibrosis and dilated bile ducts. In the infantile form, numerous small cysts (several millimeter range) develop throughout, the kidneys are markedly

enlarged, poor function is evident early on, and renal failure gradually ensues.

CT: CT reveals renal cysts to be near water density unless superimposed bleeding occurs.

MRI: Renal cysts appear rounded well-defined structures with very thin regular walls; these cysts vary from hypo- to hyperintense both with T1- and T2-weighted images, presumably due to prior hemorrhage.

- *Autosomal Dominant Polycystic Kidney Disease (ADPKD):* also called adult polycystic kidney disease and Potter type III, is the most common hereditary renal disorder. Renal failure is a late finding. These patients are also prone to developing aortic and cerebral aneurysms with their related complications.

  Clinical presentation is variable and includes dull flank pain of variable severity and time course: most common, abdominal/flank masses, hematuria, and hypertension.

  CT: CT shows most cysts to resemble simple cysts, although hemorrhage into cysts is common and these are hyperdense to water. The walls are very thin and regular and are often imperceptible. Some have a fluid–fluid level or even appear as a solid tumor. Renal calcifications are generally secondary to calculi, prior hemorrhage into a cyst, or cyst wall calcifications.

  MRI: Renal cysts appear rounded well-defined structures with very thin regular walls; these cysts vary from hypo- to hyperintense both with T1- and T2-weighted images, presumably due to prior hemorrhage.

Polycystic Ovarian Disease

- Polycystic ovarian disease (Stein–Leventhal syndrome) consists of oligomenorrhea, anovulation, hyperandrogenism, and obesity in a setting of enlarged, polycystic ovaries. Serum-luteinizing hormone levels are increased and follicle-stimulating hormone levels are decreased. Infertility is common.

- It is usually diagnosed clinically. Both ovaries are affected and may be enlarged or normal in size.
- CT: CT detects enlarged ovaries containing numerous small cysts, generally uniform in size. In some women the cysts are sufficiently small, making their identification difficult. The cysts are close to water density. Hemorrhage is rare.
- MRI: MRI reveals subcortical cysts and a thickened fibrotic capsule; with a hypointense signal from these cysts on T1- and hyperintense signal on T2-weighted images. In contrast to normal ovaries, follicles seen in polycystic ovarian disease are typically smaller than 1 cm and are uniform in size and appearance.

Polyps, Endometrial

See section "Endometrial polyp".

Prostatic Adenoma

See Chapter 2 "Benign Prostatic Hyperplasia".

Prostatic Cancer

- Prostatic cancer is one of the most frequent and most commonly diagnosed cancer in men.

- Adenocarcinoma accounts for about 95 % of all prostatic malignancies. Mucinous adenocarcinomas of the prostate are uncommon, and their prognosis is worse than that of a more typical adenocarcinoma.

  The most common initiator for a search for prostate carcinoma is a screening of an elevated PSA level. Examinations used in prostate cancer detection include digital rectal examination, transrectal US, MRI, and US-guided transrectal biopsy.
- CT: Nonhelical CT detects an enlarged gland but cannot distinguish between BPH and a neoplasm. Carcinoma is suggested only by an irregular contour outline. Helical CT, on the other hand, identified cancer in 88 % of patients as peripheral zone regions of contrast enhancement; transitional zone cancers, on the other hand, appear similar to benign nodules.
- MRI: On T2-weighted images a prostatic carcinoma typically is hypointense relative to the higher signal intensity of the normal peripheral zone. A hypointense peripheral zone is not pathognomonic for a prostatic cancer; prostatitis, benign prostatic hyperplasia, or biopsy hematoma can have a similar appearance. A wedge shape and diffuse extension without mass in a hypointense peripheral zone suggest benignity, while a large size is associated with malignancy. Cancers in the central and transitional zones are difficult to identify with MRI; when large, they tend to disrupt the normal gland architecture. Dynamic contrast-enhanced images may provide better tumor definition by outlining tumor margins more clearly than with unenhanced images. Diffusion-weighted imaging may predict the aggressivity of the cancer and is useful for detection; Fig. 7.
- 1H-MR spectroscopy reveals a correlation between water T2-relaxation time and tissue citrate concentration. Significantly higher choline levels and significantly lower citrate levels are found in cancer tissue compared with BPH and normal tissue. Men with cancer have a significantly lower citrate-to-choline ratio than those with BPH.

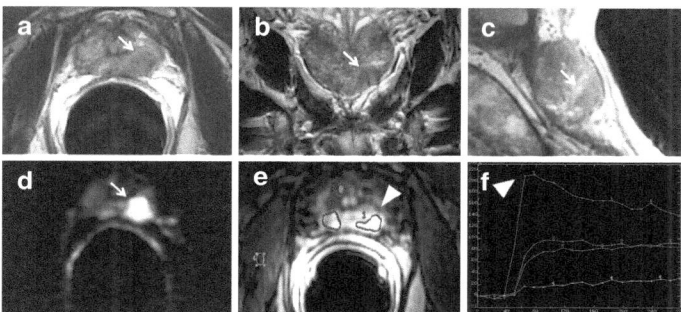

Fig. 7 An huge hypointense mass is spotted (*white arrow*) on the left part of the peripheral zone (**a**) on axial T2-weighted imaging. Sagittal and coronal scans (**b**, **c**) help to precisely locate the tumor (*white arrow*) which is in the prostate apical section. Diffusion imaging (**d**) highlights an hyperintense focus (*white arrow*) while on perfusion imaging (**e**) the single ring of interest labeled with number 1 (*arrowhead*) shows on intensity/time curve (**f**) a malignant pattern, consisting in a rapid wash-in and a delayed washout of contrast medium (*arrowhead*)

Prostatitis

- Prostatitis can be either acute or chronic. At times, a specific pathogen is detected; if not, the clinical symptoms are often ascribed to prostatodynia.
- Ultrasonography reveals a complex pattern in prostatitis.
- Early prostatic cancer and prostatitis are difficult to differentiate with current imaging.
- MRI: MRI in some patients with prostatitis MR spectroscopy detects an elevated choline peak and reduced or no citrate, mimicking cancer. Areas with prostatitis tend to enhance fast and show washout on dynamic contrast-enhanced MR imaging.

Pyelonephritis Acute

- Acute pyelonephritis (APN) primarily results from bacterial infection of the kidney by an ascending route that causes a tubulointerstitial inflammation of the renal parenchyma.
- The diagnosis is traditionally based on a combination of laboratory findings and typical clinical features, including flank pain, high-grade fever, and urinary tract infection (UTI).
- Imaging is not routinely indicated in patients with APN, and treatment, which consists of intravenous antibiotics, can be started on the basis of typical clinical and laboratory features. Situations in which imaging is indicated include exclude obstructed kidney, high-risk patients (diabetics, elderly, and immunocompromised), those with mixed clinical picture, previous renal pathology.
- TC: Typical features of acute pyelonephritis include an ill-defined, wedge-shaped area of decreased attenuation radiating from the papilla in the medulla to the cortical surface. Other findings on CT in acute pyelonephritis include focal or global enlargement of the kidney, thickening of Gerota's fascia, stranding of perinephric fat, and obliteration of perinephric fat planes. Pelvicalyceal wall thickening and enhancement secondary to ascending infection may be the only imaging feature of a kidney affected by acute pyelonephritis.
- MRI: An affected area will have low signal intensity on T1-weighted images and increased signal intensity on T2-weighted images, with a loss of normal corticomedullary differentiation. Perinephric fluid is also commonly seen but is not a specific finding for acute pyelonephritis. The use of gadolinium is essential in correctly depicting areas of renal involvement. MRI features of pyelonephritis mimic those of CT, with renal enlargement, perinephric stranding, focal areas of decreased enhancement, and striated pyelogram. Associated abscess cavities are also well seen.

Pyocele

- A pyocele consists of pus in the tunica vaginalis, generally secondary to an epididymo-orchitis or rupture of a testicular abscess.
- MRI: Abscesses are typically hypointense on T1-weighted images and hyperintense on T2-weighted images, compatible with fluid content, and T2-weighted images demonstrate a hypointense rim; on contrast-enhanced T1-weighted images, the lesion does not enhance, but the surrounding parenchyma shows avid enhancement.

Suggested Reading

Kirkham APS, Illing RO, Minhas S, et al. 2008. MR Imaging of Nonmalignant Penile Lesions, RadioGraphics 28: 837–853

Hauck EW, Hackstein N, Vosshenrich R, et al. 2003. Diagnostic Value of Magnetic Resonance Imaging in Peyronie's Disease-A Comparison Both with Palpation and Ultrasound in the Evaluation of Plaque Formation, European Urology 43: 293–300

Hase S, Mitsumori A, Inai R, et al. 2012. Endometrial polyps: MR imaging features, Acta Med Okayama 66(6): 475–85

Park SB and Lee JB. 2014. MRI Features of Ovarian Cystic Lesions, Journal of magnetic resonance imaging 00: 00–00

Tukeva TA, Aronen HJ, Karjalainen PT, et al. 1999. MR imaging in pelvic inflammatory disease: comparison with laparoscopy and US, Radiology 210: 209–216

Cassidy FH, Ishioka KM, McMahon CJ, et al. 2010. MR Imaging of Scrotal Tumors and Pseudotumors, RadioGraphics 30: 665–683

Stunell H, Buckley O, Feeney J, et al. 2007. Imaging of acute pyelonephritis in the adult, Eur Radiol 17: 1820–1828

Shukla-Dave A, Hricak H, Eberhardt SC, et al. 2004. Chronic prostatitis: MR imaging and 1H MR spectroscopic imaging findings–initial observations. Radiology;231:717–724

Prando A, Wallace S. 2000. Helical CT of prostate cancer: early clinical experience. AJR; 175:343–346

Cruz M, Tsuda K, Narumi Y, et al. 2002. Characterization of low-intensity lesions in the peripheral zone of prostate on pre-biopsy endorectal coil MR imaging.Eur Radiol;12:357–365.

Dickinson L, Ahmed HU, Allen C et al. 2013. Clinical applications of multiparametric MRI within the prostate cancer diagnostic pathway. Urol Oncol;31(3):281–4.

Q

No lemma

V. Panebianco, J.J. Fütterer, *MDCT and MRI in Genitourinary Imaging*, 109
A-Z Notes in Radiological Practice and Reporting,
DOI 10.1007/978-88-470-5705-0_17, © Springer-Verlag Italia 2015

R

Renal Adenoma

- A renal adenoma is a benign renal neoplasm. It is traditionally classified into three distinct types (renal papillary adenoma, renal tubular adenoma, and alveolar renal adenoma). The papillary type is the commonest variant with an estimated prevalence of 40 % in patients older than 70 years of age.

- Such lesions are histologically indistinguishable from larger carcinomas more commonly encountered in the kidneys, and they often have histologic grades indicating a definite potential for malignant behavior. Accordingly, most investigators believe that these lesions should be regarded as carcinomas in an early stage of evolution and should not be classified as adenomas.

- On CT, these small renal tumors are usually well defined and homogeneous in appearance. Less commonly, they show marginal irregularity, heterogeneity, or central calcification, findings that may suggest pathologically high-grade tumors. These lesions are best managed with partial nephrectomy, provided that the other kidney is normal.

V. Panebianco, J.J. Fütterer, *MDCT and MRI in Genitourinary Imaging*,   111
A-Z Notes in Radiological Practice and Reporting,
DOI 10.1007/978-88-470-5705-0_18, © Springer-Verlag Italia 2015

Renal Angiomyolipoma

- Renal angiomyolipoma (AML) is a type of benign mesenchymal neoplasm composed of adipose tissue, thick-walled vessels and smooth muscle elements in varying proportions. 80 % of angiomyolipomas are sporadic and have a female predilection (F:M of 4:1). 20 % can be seen in association with phakomatoses, e.g., tuberous sclerosis, and in these cases they present earlier, are larger and far more numerous.
- When they are symptomatic, they present with spontaneous retroperitoneal hemorrhage. The bleeding risk is proportional to the size of the lesion, being greater if it measures more than 4 cm. Other common signs and symptoms are palpable mass, flank pain, urinary tract infections, hematuria, renal failure, and hypertension.
- When the triad of adipose tissue, thick-walled vessels, and smooth muscle elements is present, the radiologic diagnosis is uncomplicated. However, "monophasic" variants exist, i.e., consisting of only one of these three components, such as the form composed exclusively of spindle-shaped smooth muscle cells, or the epithelioid variant, which is particularly problematic because it can be interpreted as a carcinoma.
- On CT, most lesions involve the cortex and demonstrate macroscopic fat (<20 HU). Sometimes, especially in the context of a syndrome, they can be fat-poor.
- MRI is a valuable tool at evaluating fat-containing lesions, and two main set of sequences are employed, that is fat saturated techniques (which demonstrate high signal on nonfat saturated sequences, and loss of signal following fat saturation) and in and out of phase imaging which generates India ink artifact at the interface between fat and nonfat components. It is important to remember that rarely renal cell carcinomas may have macroscopic fat components; therefore, the presence of fat is suggestive of an angiomyolipoma, but it is not pathognomonic.

Renal Bacterial Infection (Acute Pyelonephritis)

- Pyelonephritis is an infectious process affecting the kidney, which is caused mainly by Gram-negative bacteria (*E. coli*, *Proteus*, *Pseudomonas*, *Klebsiella*, and *Enterococcus* species), whereas less than 20 % of cases are caused by Gram-positive bacteria. Ascending infections caused by bacteria of the fecal flora are the most common, especially in patients with concomitant urinary tract diseases such as lithiasis or vesicoureteric.

- Acute pyelonephritis can be defined as a clinical syndrome characterized by lumbar pain and hyperpyrexia, associated with laboratory findings of renal bacterial infection including leukocytosis, pyuria, bacteriuria, and positive urine culture. In anatomopathologic terms, pyelonephritis is a bacterial infection of the kidney, with consequent acute inflammation often involving the pelvis and renal parenchyma of both kidneys. This causes suppurative interstitial inflammation with tubular necrosis.

- Imaging is needed to determine if there are complications requiring prolonged antibiotic therapy or surgical intervention (e.g., renal and perinephric abscess or pyonephrosis). Imaging is also useful for excluding abnormalities that predispose to refractory infections such as nephrolithiasis or ureteral obstruction.

- In patients with acute bacterial renal infection, CT scans are acquired with contrast enhancement during the corticomedullary phase (30 s after initiation of injection) and during either the nephrographic phase (70–90 s after injection) or the excretory phase (5 min after injection). A nephrogram on contrast-enhanced CT that consists of discrete rays of alternating attenuation extending to the cortex is characteristic of pyelonephritis and is better demonstrated on CT than on excretory urography. Striations result from stasis of contrast material within edematous tubules that demonstrates increasing attenuation over time. Severe tubulointerstitial inflammation may progress to form a hypodense mass or masses with rounded or irregular contours and bulging of the renal surface. If treated too late or inadequately, such lesions may develop single or multiple small areas of liquefaction (i.e., small abscesses). These areas are often irregular and of near water attenuation (20–30 HU); they do not enhance after intravenous administration of contrast medium.

Renal Cell Carcinoma

- The most common renal cancer is the carcinoma (renal cell carcinoma, RCC), which accounts for 3 % of all adult cancers and 80–85 % of malignant renal tumors.
- Patients with RCC can present with a range of symptoms; unfortunately, many patients are asymptomatic until the disease is advanced. At presentation, approximately 25 % of individuals either have distant metastases or advanced locoregional disease. The classic triad of RCC (flank pain, hematuria, and a palpable abdominal renal mass) occurs in most 9 % of patients. Many patients with RCC present with or subsequently develop systemic symptoms or paraneoplastic syndromes.
- Of all the available prognostic factors, tumor extension at diagnosis is the most important element for predicting disease progression; as a result, CT plays a key role and still today can be considered the best imaging modality for staging RCC.
- CT is currently recognized as the best imaging technique for *identifying* renal parenchymal neoplasms. CT can identify more and smaller lesions than US, although it is unable to improve on their characterization; Fig. 8. There are two fundamental aims to the *characterization* of solid renal lesions to distinguish a renal tumor from normal anatomic variants or

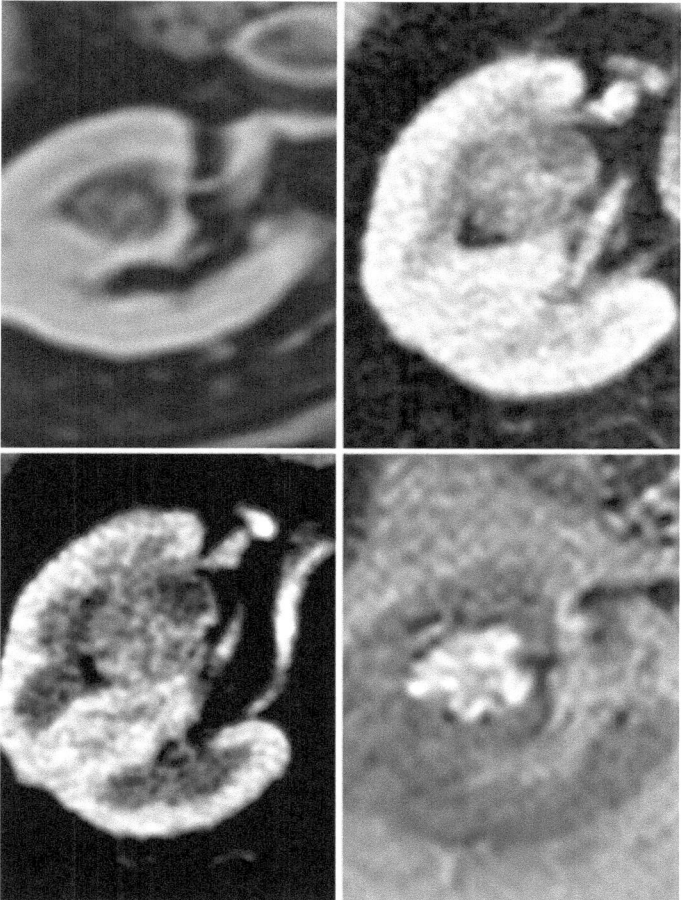

Fig. 8 CT images showing a capsulated renal mass with inhomogeneous contrast enhancement on arterial and venous phase which was found to be a Renal Cell Carcinoma. MR images depicting a round-shaped, well-capsulated renal mass with inhomogeneous high signal intensity on T2-weighted images and contrast enhancement, without any signs of infiltration of renal vein. After surgery this mass was found to be a Renal Cell Carcinoma

thrombus into the vena cava itself, where it becomes evident as an intraluminal defect. CT remains the most immediately used imaging modality for the evaluation of distant metastases (lungs, liver, and skeletal system). The most specific CT parameter for classifying a solid mass as T3a is provided by the identification of a solid enhancing nodule in the perirenal fat, which possibly behaves in a similar manner to the primary lesion. Stranding and increased thickness of perirenal fat are not necessarily signs of tumor spread, since they are identifiable in 50 % of patients with lesions confined to the capsule.

- MRI has an important role to play in the characterization of renal lesions. Thanks to the efficacy of the dynamic study, the increase in signal intensity can be measured over time and the vasculature of small lesions can be evaluated. In T1-weighted images medium to large lesions can appear hypo-isointense or even weakly (but never clearly) hyperintense. In T2-weighted sequences, the appearance is hypo- and hyperintense. MR is able to resolve the problems CT has with complex cysts, i.e., small lesions with calcified walls, in which the absence of enhancement can help make the diagnosis of benign lesions.

Renal Cysts (Simple Renal Cyst)

- The most common causes of radiologically evident renal cysts in adults are simple renal cysts, which will be discussed here, autosomal dominant polycystic kidney disease, and, acquired cystic disease in patients with end-stage renal disease after several years of dialysis, particularly hemodialysis. Unusual causes of renal cysts in adults are Von Hippel–Lindau disease, tuberous sclerosis complex, and nephronophthisis. Postmortem studies have shown that more than 50 % of people under the age of 50 have one or more cysts.

- To help diagnose and manage these lesions, the Bosniak renal cyst classification system was created. Based upon morphologic and enhancement characteristics with CT scanning, cystic renal masses are placed into one of five different categories. The presence of true contrast enhancement of the lesion (a minimum increased attenuation of 10–15 Hounsfield units) is the most important characteristic separating categories III and IV, which are associated with malignancy in 40–90 %, from the categories I, II, and IIF, which are typically benign processes.
- MRI is typically used to evaluate patients with indeterminate lesions. In addition to signal characteristics, MRI evaluates the same morphologic findings as described above for CT scanning: wall thickening, nodularity, septa, and enhancement. One difference is that MRI does not detect calcification. MRI is especially useful for characterizing internal contents of cysts, such as hemorrhage or mucin, and is more sensitive than both ultrasonography and CT in showing enhancement of internal septations. The combination of mural irregularity and intense mural enhancement had the highest correlation with malignancy.

  Serial MRI examinations at 3, 6, and 12 months are warranted in patients with indeterminate lesions on gadolinium-enhanced MRI.

Renal Lipomatosis

- Renal sinus lipomatosis refers to a condition where there is excessive renal sinus fat replacement, which can be due to inflammation, renal parenchymal atrophy, renal stones, ageing or steroids.
- There is a variant, called "replacement lipomatosis of the kidney" in which infection, renal calculi, and long-standing hydronephrosis are accompanied by severe renal parenchymal damage.

- Minor anatomic variants like this one are commonly encountered and are usually evaluated using excretory urography. However, CT is sometimes necessary for further evaluation when urographic findings are confusing. Renal sinus lipomatosis may masquerade as mass lesion in the renal sinus, but CT reveals the benign nature of the process by showing that the renal sinus is occupied by tissue with a fat-attenuation value.

Renal Medullary Carcinoma

- Renal medullary carcinoma is a rare tumor of the kidney. This tumor occurs exclusively in young black patients with sickle cell trait (HbSA and HbSC) but not sickle cell anemia. Affected patients range from 11 to 39 years in age.
- Flank pain and hematuria are the most common presenting symptoms. Metastatic involvement of regional lymph nodes, liver, and lungs at presentation is common.
- The radiologic appearance of renal medullary carcinoma is that of a prototypical infiltrative lesion. An ill-defined mass centered in the renal medulla with extension into the renal sinus and cortex is characteristic; caliectasis may be seen, and the reniform contour of the kidney is maintained. The tumors are heterogeneous on ultrasonography and contrast-enhanced CT, reflecting the characteristic tumor necrosis. The prognosis is extremely poor. The constellation of renal medullary mass, black race, sickle cell trait, and hemoglobin SC disease suggests the diagnosis.

Renal Pelvis, Transitional Cell Carcinoma of

- Transitional cell carcinoma (TCC) of the renal pelvis is an uncommon cancer, and it can be challenging to identify on routine imaging. Renal pelvis tumors are more common in males, and are typically diagnosed during the sixth decade.

- Microscopic or macroscopic hematuria is the typical present-ing symptom. Depending on the location, symptomatic hydronephrosis may be the presenting symptom (flank pain) and a renal colic due to a clot may mimic an impacted calcu-lus. Patients may also present once metastatic disease becomes symptomatic.

- CT urographic study is performed in two or more dynamic phases. An initial baseline examination to rule out stone for-mations is followed by a delayed arterial or early corticome-dullary phase acquired 15–25 s after the injection of contrast medium, which is especially useful in identifying vascular anomalies. The nephrographic phase used for the study of the renal parenchyma begins at 80–140 s after the injection of contrast medium. The final excretory phase is acquired at 4–8 min and enables study of the collecting system and the bladder. TCCs ≥ 1 cm can be visualized in the baseline exam-ination as solid or cystic-like lesions with attenuation values between 8 and 40 HU, location in the renal pelvis or a calyx, and a round, plaque-like or arborescent appearance. In the arterial and venous phases of the dynamic study, there is a moderate but significant increase in the attenuation values of the lesion. TCC is identified in the excretory phase as a ses-sile, nodular filling defect with lobulated margins. Occasionally dilatation of a calyx, hydronephrosis, and/or delayed enhancement of the collecting system may be the only signs of the presence of a lesion. When the tumor is invasive, its extraluminal growth can be identified with inva-sion of the perirenal pelvic fat and/or psoas muscle. In addi-tion, multidetector-row CT is able to study its precise anatomy and relations with the arterial and venous vessels. The dif-ferential diagnosis should include pelvicalyceal inflamma-tory processes, which can produce wall thickening and heterogeneity of the surrounding adipose tissue.

- MR urography is especially indicated in children, pregnancy, and patients with known allergies to iodinated contrast medium. The study can be either static or dynamic. Static examination is done with heavily T2-weighted images to exploit the hyperintense signal of the static or semistationary fluids such as urine in the event of stenosis of the collecting system. Dynamic study can be done with or without an associated diuretic agent and is performed after the injection of gadolinium, which is concentrated in the collecting system during the delayed phase. Like on CT images, tumors of the pelvicaliceal cavities appear on MR urography as filling defects with a vegetative polypoid appearance and irregular or stippled margins. Their attachment, which is readily identifiable at the level of the pelvis, is more challenging in lesions arising from the calices or collecting ducts due to the limited size of their lumina. TCC appears isointense to renal parenchyma in T1- and T2-weighted images, and hypointense to urine in T2-weighted images, making its identification simple in the event of dilatation of the pelvicalyceal cavity. Despite being hypovascular, the lesion may appear moderately enhancing after contrast medium administration.

Renal Sinus Cyst

- Renal sinus cysts (parapelvic) are benign extraparenchymal cysts located in the renal sinus. They are not true renal cysts but are probably lymphatic in origin. They may be unilocular or multilocular and are often bilateral. They do not communicate with the renal collecting system.
- Most renal sinus cysts are asymptomatic and are discovered incidentally on imaging studies. They may in rare cases cause hypertension, hematuria, and hydronephrosis, or may become secondarily infected.

- Renal sinus cysts display the same CT features as simple renal parenchymal cysts. They have attenuation values in the water range and are difficult to distinguish from dilated or extrarenal renal pelvis on unenhanced CT scans. The characteristic feature of a sinus renal cyst is a surrounding halo of renal sinus fat, indicating its extrarenal origin. After intravenous administration of contrast medium, the cysts remain of water density and cause displacement of the renal pelvis and calyces. Differentiation from hydronephrosis is thus readily made on contrast-enhanced CT. CT easily distinguishes between renal sinus cyst and renal sinus lipomatosis, which causes a similar deformity of the collecting system on excretory urography. In renal sinus lipomatosis, the attenuation value of the tissue is in the fat range. Solid masses in the renal sinus, such as lymphoma and invasive transitional cell carcinoma, are readily differentiated from renal sinus cyst because of their soft tissue attenuation values.

Renal Transplantation

- Renal transplantation makes the recipients susceptible to a number of complications. These can be broadly categorized as perirenal, renal parenchymal (acute and chronic rejection), renal collecting system (urinoma), and renal vascular complication (renal artery stenosis and renal vein thrombosis). Complications not confined to the kidney are avascular necrosis, amyloidosis, metastatic joint calcification, and increased incidence of malignancy (especially hematologic malignancy).
- Radiologic evaluation for suspected surgical complications and of kidney dysfunction in patients with renal transplants is best achieved by renal scintigraphy and ultrasonography. Peritransplant fluid collections, including hematomas,

lymphoceles, abscesses, and urinomas, are readily assessed on ultrasonography. Unenhanced CT and MRI are reserved for cases in which ultrasonography fails either because of lack of access due to a recent surgical incision or because the transplant area is obscured by intestinal gas. Contrast-enhanced CT should be avoided because of the potential for nephrotoxicity. MRI is a suitable alternative in the evaluation of the transplanted kidney and peritransplant region; however, sonography and sonographic-guided biopsy remain the primary imaging and interventional modalities.

Renal Vein, Diseases of

- Renal vein occlusions may be categorized into five groups: (1) extrinsic occlusion of the renal vein by an adjacent neoplasm; (2) direct renal vein extension of RCC or adrenal neoplasms; (3) renal vein thrombosis associated with primary renal disease (e.g., about 20 % of patients with the nephrotic syndrome); (4) secondary renal vein occlusion or thrombosis may occur when the inferior vena cava is thrombosed after caval extension of thrombus from pelvic or leg veins; and (5) renal vein thrombosis, which may occur as a primary phenomenon.
- A classic acute presentation consists of flank pain, hematuria, and loss of renal function. Patients with chronic renal vein occlusion are usually asymptomatic.
- Contrast-enhanced CT is an excellent method for the noninvasive diagnosis of renal vein thrombosis, provided that renal function is normal. CT permits differentiation between acute renal vein thrombosis and conditions that have similar clinical presentations, such as acute pyelonephritis, acute renal infarction, and acute renal obstruction. Renal vein thrombosis

is generally unilateral. In acute and subacute cases, an enlarged, swollen kidney is seen on CT. The nephrogram in the affected kidney is initially diminished because of impaired renal perfusion; however, once the nephrogram develops, it persists for a prolonged period and there is often prolonged enhancement of the renal cortex relative to the renal medulla. Calyceal opacification is often delayed, diminished, or absent in the affected kidney. Stranding of the perinephric fat due to edema and thickening of the renal fascia may occur. Enlarged perirenal collateral veins are often noted. Perinephric hemorrhage may occur. On CT, the renal vein is commonly enlarged and may show a filling defect because of thrombus. Thrombosis of the inferior vena cava at *or* near the renal vein orifices occurs in about 40–50 % of patients with renal vein thrombosis. Demonstration of venous thrombus is facilitated by scanning during the peak phase of vascular opacification after bolus injection of contrast medium and by obtaining 5-mm-thick sections.

- MRI is widely used for detecting renal vein extension of RCC; it can also be used in the evaluation of nonneoplastic renal vein thrombosis. MRI is most useful for evaluating patients with significant renal functional impairment and symptoms suggesting renal vein thrombosis. Renal vein thrombus may be shown on T1-weighted spin-echo pulse sequences when the signal void of flowing blood in the renal vein is replaced by high signal because of thrombus. Gradient-echo technique shows thrombus as a filling defect of medium signal intensity that replaces the high signal of flowing blood. Coronal MRI helps determine the extent of involvement in the vena cava. MRI in patients with acute renal vein thrombosis may also show loss of corticomedullary differentiation on T1-weighted spin-echo images, increased signal in the affected kidney on T2-weighted images, renal fascial thickening, and renal enlargement.

Renal Oncocytoma

- Renal oncocytoma is a rare benign renal tumor, but it is clinically important since distinguishing it preoperatively from renal cell carcinoma (which has similar epidemiology, presentation, imaging, and even histology) may be particularly challenging. Renal oncocytomas account for only 5 % of resected primary adult epithelial renal neoplasms. They typically present during the 6th or 7th decade, similar to renal cell carcinoma.
- On CT, oncocytomas typically are well-defined masses with smooth, rounded margins. Tumor calcification occurs rarely, and oncocytomas are sometimes multiple and bilateral. Small oncocytomas are usually homogeneous in appearance on contrast-enhanced CT scans, although they are occasionally heterogeneous because of the presence of central scars. On CT, small oncocytomas are usually indistinguishable from slowly growing small RCCs that lack hemorrhage or necrosis. A central, sharply defined stellate scar is present in up to one-third of large oncocytomas and strongly suggests the diagnosis. However, CT criteria are usually poor discriminants for distinguishing between oncocytoma and RCC, regardless of tumor size.
- On MRI, oncocytoma is generally isointense to hypointense to normal parenchyma on T1-weighted images and has a variable appearance on T2-weighted images (it may be hyperintense compared to renal cortex and may demonstrate hypointense central renal scar, which suggests the diagnosis). Oncocytomas do enhance in a homogeneous fashion with gadolinium administration, but less than renal parenchyma.

Renal Trauma

- Renal trauma may be caused by both blunt and penetrating abdominal injuries. Blunt trauma is responsible for most renal injuries. Such injuries are usually mild and heal without specific therapy. Serious renal injury is often associated with damage to other structures.

- Renal injuries are classified into four categories on the basis of imaging findings. Category I lesions (75–85 % of cases) are clinically insignificant; they consist of contusions and small corticomedullary lacerations that do not communicate with the collecting system. Category II lesions (10 % of cases) are more serious and comprise major lacerations through the renal cortex extending to the medulla or collecting systems with or without urinary extravasation. Category III lesions (5 % of cases), which are catastrophic, consist of shattered kidney (multiple deep lacerations) and injury to the renal pedicle. The rare entities of ureteropelvic junction avulsion and laceration of the renal pelvis are designated as category IV lesions.
- Gross hematuria is the most reliable indication of potentially serious renal damage. However, the absence of hematuria does not preclude significant renal injury.
- Contrast-enhanced CT is the preferred modality for evaluation of patients with blunt or penetrating abdominal trauma with scans obtained at 70 s and 3 min after the start of injection of contrast material. The three basic types of renal injury demonstrable by CT are contusions, lacerations, and infarcts, any of which may be further complicated by intrarenal or extrarenal hematomas or by urinary extravasation. The mildest form of renal injury is the contusion, characterized by an amorphous, interstitial extravasation of blood and edema. On unenhanced CT scans, the affected kidney zones may show focal swelling and irregular infiltrates of high-density fresh blood. On contrast-enhanced CT, renal contusions appear as ill-defined, round or ovoid areas of hypoattenuation. Superficial lacerations are limited to the renal cortex; deep lacerations extend into the medulla, where they may enter the collecting system or transect the kidney. Contrast extravasation

is often seen in the perinephric space. In patients with multiple lacerations (shattered kidney), the fragments are separated and surrounded by blood clot. Thrombosis or laceration of a segmental branch of the renal artery produces a focal area of renal infarction. Infarcts typically appear as peripherally based, wedge-shaped areas of parenchyma that fail to enhance during both the corticomedullary and pyelographic phases of CT. Posttraumatic bleeding is commonly associated with all injuries to the kidney. Hematomas may be intrarenal or sub-capsular or may involve the perinephric or pararenal spaces. The most significant vascular injury after blunt trauma is thrombosis of the main renal artery; the diagnosis of pedicle injury can be suggested by a hematoma surrounding the renal hilus and abrupt cutoff of the contrast-filled renal artery. Acute renal vein occlusion may be suspected if the kidney is enlarged and shows thrombus in the renal vein. Ureteropelvic junction injuries are rare. In these patients, CT typically dem-onstrates excellent excretion of contrast material with an intact intrarenal collecting system, but with medial perineph-ric urinary extravasation rather than lateral urinary extravasa-tion in category II injuries with involvement of the collecting system. A circumrenal urinoma may be seen around the affected kidney, but typically, there is no perinephric hematoma.

- Gadolinium-enhanced MRI may be used to assess suspected renal injury when the use of iodinated contrast material is contraindicated.

Reninoma

- Renin-producing tumors (juxtaglomerular neoplasm or reni-nomas) are a rare, but curable, cause of hypertension. Two-thirds of juxtaglomerular cell tumors of the kidney occur in young women of child-bearing age. None of the reported neoplasms has been invasive or has metastasized.

- Reninomas are usually well shown on contrast-enhanced CT scans on which they show a smooth outline and sharp margination. Small foci of hemorrhage may cause a heterogeneous tumor appearance. Because of their benign nature, reninomas may be managed by partial nephrectomy.
- On MRI, reninomas are isointense to hypointense to normal cortex on TI-weighted images and hypointense to normal cortex on T2-weighted images. These tumors tend to enhance less than normal cortex on MRI because of their relative hypovascular architecture.

Retroperitoneal Fibrosis

- Retroperitoneal fibrosis is a proliferation of fibrous and/or chronic inflammatory tissue in the retroperitoneum. Its incidence is 1:200000, it is three times more common in men, and the peak incidence is in the 6th decade. It can be primary or secondary.
- Symptoms are nonspecific: diffuse, dull back pain; weight loss, leg lymphedema.
- The modality of choice to investigate this condition is MRI, and US can then be used for follow-up. Pathognomonic findings are proliferation of fibrous tissue in the retroperitoneal space, fibrotic process surrounding the aorta and ureters, medial deviation of the mid-ureters, and concentric ureteral narrowing.
- On MRI, there is retroperitoneal proliferation of fibrous tissue that may extend from the pelvic wall to the renal hilum. The tissue has low signal intensity on T1-weighted images and moderately low signal intensity on T2-weighted images. Encasement of the aorta and ureters is often evident. If there

is an acute inflammatory process, this will be indicated by increased signal intensity on T2-weighted images and more marked enhancement. Medial deviation of the ureters is sometimes observed and there is possible urinary obstruction. Thickening and irregularity of the aortic wall is often associated with idiopathic retroperitoneal fibrosis. A highly inhomogeneous appearance on T2-weighted images suggests the malignant form of retroperitoneal fibrosis.

• On CT, there is low-attenuating fibrous tissue in the retroperitoneum. The other findings are similar to those on MRI. Differential diagnosis should include urothelial carcinoma of the ureter and retroperitoneal lymphadenopathy.

Retroperitoneum in Renal Cell Carcinoma, Bladder Cancer, and Other Pelvic Neoplasms

• Retroperitoneal lymph node enlargement can be encountered in patients with renal cell carcinoma (RCC). Both CT and MRI appear equally effective in detecting retroperitoneal lymph node metastases, but these techniques are usually helpful only when bulky metastatic disease is present. Unfortunately, RCC and other pelvic malignancies frequently metastasize to normal sized or only slightly enlarged nodes, so that identification of tumor spread to pelvic and retroperitoneal nodes by CT and MRI is often impossible. Reported sensitivities for detecting abdominal and pelvic lymph node involvement vary widely, and specificities have also been less than optimal. Some work has demonstrated that MRI lymph node enhancement with gadolinium-based contrast material is more rapid when metastases from bladder cancer are present. This difference in enhancement rate between normal and abnormal lymph nodes has resulted in MRI detection of metastatic disease even in normal-sized lymph nodes. On CT scan, however, lymph nodes invaded with metastatic tumor occasionally enhance with contrast material to the same extent as adjacent vessels. Such enhancement, which has been observed in some patients with bladder cancer and some other nonpelvic primary neoplasms (e.g., thyroid and RCC), may lead to the erroneous impression that lymph nodes actually represent abnormal dilated vessels.

Suggested Reading

Israel GM, Bosniak MA. 2005. An update of the Bosniak renal cyst classification system. Urology; 66:484

Balci NC, Semelka RC, Patt RH, et al. 1999. Complex renal cysts: findings on MR imaging. AJR Am J Roentgenol; 172:1495.

Vivas I, Nicolás AI, Velázquez P et al. 2000. Retroperitoneal fibrosis: typical and atypical manifestations. Br J Radiol; 73: 214–222

Arancibia MF, Bolenz C, Michel MS et al. 2007. The modern management of upper tract urothelial cancer: surgical treatment. BJU Int; 99:978–981

Israel GM, Hindman N, Hecht E et al. 2005. The use of opposed-phase chemical shift MRI in the diagnosis of renal angiomyolipomas. AJR Am J Roentgenol; 184:1868–72

Browne RF, Meehan CO, Colville J et al. 2005 Transitional cell carcinoma of the upper urinary tract: spectrum of imaging findings. RadioGraphics; 25:1609–1627

S

Sarcoidosis of Genitourinary Tract

- Sarcoidosis is considered a multisystem disorder of unclear etiology which can affect many organ, characterized by the presence of widespread, noncaseating granulomas. It is thought to represent a disorder of cell-mediated immunity. It presents a wide spectrum of clinical manifestations and radiographic findings.
- Renal involvement is seen in 8–19 % of patients; sarcoidosis may occasionally have a pseudotumors (lymphoma or metastases) appearance with multiple hypodense lesions involving both kidneys. Their similar enhancement to the rest of the kidney on CT or MRI distinguishes them from malignant lesions. The lesion does not usually distort the renal margin. Characteristically, there is central extension of the column of Bertin. Hydronephrosis may be caused by compression of the ureters by enlarged retroperitoneal nodes.
- Testicular sarcoidosis has been found in 5 % of patients at autopsy. Testicular sarcoidosis presents with a unilateral, nodular, painless scrotal mass in young males. US is the gold standard; in equivocal cases of epididymal involvement,

T2-weighted MRI may reveal a high signal intensity area on a background of normal epididymal tissue.

Sedation for Image-Guided Microsurgery

• Two types of medication may be given to patients: one for sedation and anxiety, a mild sedative such as Midazolam, and another for analgesia. In most average-size adult patients, 1 mg intravenously can be given at the onset and then titrate the needs of the patient during the procedure. As a rule it is probably better to err on the side of giving medication, but if there is no apparent need by the history or from clinical observation of the patient, one should withhold the drugs.

Scrotal Hernia

• Diagnosis of scrotal hernia is usually made on clinically findings, but in rare cases (i.e., patient size, marked enlargement of the scrotum accompanied by acute testicular pain) should be used Magnetic Resonance.
• MRI demonstrates a complex masse within the scrotum and adjacent normal testicular tissue. MRI findings could include air within the bowel or fat content of the mesentery, meconium hernia misdiagnosed on US as testicular mass.

Scrotal Trauma

• Patients present with an acute scrotum and history of trauma. Diagnosis is made in combination with clinical history and US findings.

- MRI can be a useful alternative diagnostic modality for blunt scrotal trauma, especially when ultrasonography results in an inconclusive diagnosis; interruption of the dark signal intensity line of the tunica albuginea being pathognomonic for the diagnosis of testicular rupture.

Seminal Vesicle Cyst

- The seminal vesicles are easily identified on MR images as convoluted tubular structures coursing posterior and superior to the base of the prostate. The seminal fluid shows high signal intensity on T2-weighted images. The walls show low signal intensity.
- Because of spread of tumor to the seminal vesicle occurs directly from the base of the gland or via the ejaculatory ducts, it is important to image the inferior aspect of the seminal vesicle separately from the (low signal intensity) base of the gland with coronal sagittal images.
- Seminal vesicle invasion of prostatic carcinoma has been categorized into three types on the basis of pathologic studies of prostatectomy specimens.

  - Type 1: The most common, invasion involve extension along the ejaculatory ducts superiorly into the medial aspect of the seminal vesicles or ampullae of the vas deferens.
  - Type 2: Invasion involves direct growth superiorly from the base of the prostate into the periprostatic tissue and then into the seminal vesicles.
  - Type 3: Invasion involves foci of tumor within the seminal vesicle without evident connection to tumor in the prostate. These foci may represent metastases.

Suggested Reading

Wheeler TM. 1989. Anatomic considerations in carcinoma of the prostate. Urol clin north am 16:623–634.

Kodama K, Hasegawa T, Egawa M, et al. 2004. Bilateral epididymal sarcoidosis presenting without radiographic evidence of intrathoracic lesion: review of sarcoidosis involving the male reproductive tract. Int J Urol;11:345–348

Warshauer DM, Lee JK. 2004. Imaging manifestations of abdominal sarcoidosis. AJR Am J Roentgenol. 2004;182 (1): 15–28.

Schnall MD, Bezzi M, Pollack HM, et al. 1990. Magnetic resonance imaging of the prostate. Magn Reson Q 6:1–16.

Parivar F, Waluch V. 1992. Magnetic resonance imaging of prostate cancer. Hum pathol 23:335–343.

Hricak H, Carrington BM. 1992. MRI of the Pelvis: A Text Atlas

Miller BH, Rosado-de-christenson ML, Mcadams HP et al. 1995. Thoracic sarcoidosis: radiologic-pathologic correlation. Radiographics;15 (2): 421–37.

Kim SH, Park S, Choi SH, et al. 2009. The efficacy of magnetic resonance imaging for the diagnosis of testicular rupture: a prospective preliminary study. J Trauma;66(1):239–42

T

Testicular Cancer

- It can be divided into primary tumors and secondary tumors (lymphoma, leukemia, and metastasis). Primary tumors can be also classified into testicular germ-cell tumors and testicular nongerm-cell tumors. MR imaging is an important imaging tool in the evaluation of scrotal masses, in addition to ultrasound.
- Most intratesticular solid masses represent malignant tumors, whereas 97 % of the extratesticular masses are benign.

Germ-Cell Tumors (95 % of Testicular Carcinomas)

- They are categorized as seminoma or nonseminomatous tumor. Nonseminomatous germ-cell tumors include embryonal carcinoma, yolk sac tumor, teratoma, and choriocarcinoma.
- US is the best diagnostic tool to identify and characterize scrotal mass. Seminomas tend to be homogeneous in echotexture, whereas nonseminomatous germ-cell tumors are more heterogeneous. CT is the study of choice for the evaluation of retroperitoneal adenopathies and lung metastasis.

V. Panebianco, J.J. Fütterer, *MDCT and MRI in Genitourinary Imaging*,   135
A-Z Notes in Radiological Practice and Reporting,
DOI 10.1007/978-88-470-5705-0_20, © Springer-Verlag Italia 2015

- Seminomas are isointense to normal tissue on T1- and hypointense and homogeneous on T2-weighted MR images compared to normal testis; they enhance less than normal testicular tissue. Nonseminomatous tumors are more heterogeneous than seminomas in all MRI sequences, as they contain areas of high and low signal intensity both with T1- and T2-weighted images.

Nongerm-Cell Tumors

- Nongerm-cell tumors include Leydig cell tumor, Sertoli cell tumor, and granulosa cell tumor. Most of these tumors are benign; combinations of several of these tumors can also occur.
- The most common nongerm-cell tumor is Leydig cell tumor. It is usually well-marginated, encapsulated, solid and homogenous mass, sometimes difficult to differentiate from germ-cell tumors, in particular from seminoma. It is isointense on T1-weighted images and hypointense on T2-weighted images; in some cases, it can contain foci of increased signal intensity both on T1- and T2-weighted images.

Testicular Torsion

- The acute scrotum often presents as pain, swelling, or a combination of sudden onset. It can occur at all ages of childhood, but with two peaks: one in the newborns and the other during puberty. It consists of a twisting of testis and spermatic cord within scrotum; it causes acute scrotal pain because of vascular occlusion and infarction. Torsion of the testicular appendage should be suspected in younger boys. The role of ultrasound in the acute scrotum is to narrow the differential diagnosis to allow conservative management or expedite surgery. US is the imaging modality of choice. With acute torsion, MRI may demonstrate a twisting spermatic cord, called whirlpool sign, with a hypointense signal. Testis appears heterogeneous on all image sequences. Enhancement is low if blood flow is compromised, whereas enhancement could be very intense if detorsion has occurred.

Transplantation of Kidney

Pretransplant Evaluation

- CT allows assessment of the feasibility of kidney transplantation.
- CT provides a wide range of information regarding the vascular and extravascular systems. For example, multiple arteries can complicate kidney transplantation and may cause postoperative bleeding; the surgeon must preserve each multiple arteries to save the renal segment.
- MRI and MRA are useful to detect accessory renal arteries, some anomalous draining renal and also urinary collecting system abnormalities in living renal donors.

Posttransplant Evaluation

- In case of rejection, at MR imaging, corticomedullary differentiation tends to be preserved in acute tubular necrosis and disrupted in rejection. It occurs immediately after transplantation and it generally resolvers in 2 weeks. CT demonstrates decreased graft enhancement with no contrast material excretion. Chronic rejection can occur after months or even years after surgery and is due to sclerosing vasculitis and extensive interstitial fibrosis; allograft is usually small, often calcified.
- CT and MRI can also detect posttransplant complications such as vascular complications (arterial stenosis, thrombosis, and vein occlusion), fluid collections, ureter complications, infections, and neoplasm.

Tuberculosis, Kidney

- Renal infection results from hematogenous spread at the time of primary infection, initially both kidneys are infected, but generally the disease progresses unilaterally. Typically the papillae are involved first, then cortical damage occurs.
- At the beginning, it develops a local infection (tuberculoma), which is hypointense on both T1- and T2-weighted images, whereas on CT it is seen as a solid mass with minimal enhancement after contrast administration. Tuberculoma can resolve or enlarge and become necrotic, extending to collecting systems.
- Imaging at this stage reveals parenchymal destruction, fibrosis, scarring of the collecting system, strictures of the collecting system and of the ureteres.
- An end-stage tuberculosis kidney appears as a small, completely calcified kidney; this aspect is called "putty kidney", referring to the pattern of caseous necrosis associated with calcifications.

Suggested Reading

Perla SB, Ch S. 2012. Bilateral Multiple Renal Arteries-An Anatomical Study. WebmedCentral Anatomy;3(6):WMC003493

Sebastià C, Quiroga S, Boyé R et-al. 2001. Helical CT in renal transplantation: normal findings and early and late complications. Radiographics. 21 (5): 1103–17.

Jha RC, Korangy SJ, Ascher SM, et al. 2002. MR angiography and preoperative evaluation for laparoscopic donor nephrectomy. AJR; 178:1489–1495.

Fink C, Hallscheidt PJ, Hosch WP, et al. 2003. Preoperative evaluation of living renal donors: value of contrast- enhanced 3D magnetic resonance angiography and comparison of three rendering algorithms. Eur Radiol;13:794–801.

Sohaib SA, Koh DM, Husband JE. 2008. The role of imaging in the diagnosis, staging, and management of testicular cancer. AJR Am J Roentgenol;191 (2): 387–95.

Merchant S, Bharati A, Merchant N. 2013. Tuberculosis of the genito-urinary system-Urinary tract tuberculosis: Renal tuberculosis-Part II. Indian J Radiol Imaging;23:64–77

U

Ureter, Circumcaval

- Occasionally, an abnormally positioned IVC or a periureteric venous ring at the level of the third or fourth lumbar vertebral body medially displaces the right ureter. This abnormality, termed the circumcaval (or retrocaval) ureter, occurs with a frequency of approximately 0.1 %.
- It results from anomalous development of the infrarenal vena cava.
- In general, patients are asymptomatic. Symptoms (secondary to obstruction), when present, usually appear late.
- CT and MRI can be used to identify a circumcaval ureter if the right ureter partially encircles the inferior cava, passing first posteriorly and then medially to the IVC. Lateral positioning of the upper abdominal IVC in relation to the right ureter without an identifiable retrocaval component of the ureter, although seen in all patients with circumcaval ureters, is usually a normal variant (6 % of the general population).

V. Panebianco, J.J. Fütterer, *MDCT and MRI in Genitourinary Imaging*, 141
A-Z Notes in Radiological Practice and Reporting,
DOI 10.1007/978-88-470-5705-0_21, © Springer-Verlag Italia 2015

Ureter, Ectopic

- The incidence of ureteral ectopia is 1:1,900. It is most common in female with a marked prevalence (female:male of 5–6:1). Around 10 % of ureteral ectopias are bilateral.
- An ectopic ureter is one that drains in an abnormal location (outside the posterolateral angle of the trigone) either within the bladder (intravesical) or extravesically. Vesicoureteric reflux is often associated, although the condition may be asymptomatic. Ectopic ureter, however, more commonly refers to the extravesical form and is clinically more important than the intravesical type.
- Extravesical ureteral ectopia in females is associated with a duplicated system in at least 85 % of cases and affects the upper pole ureter in practically all cases. The ectopic ureter may end in the urethra or in the vestibule or, less commonly, in the vagina.
- Ultrasound is the imaging modality of choice and often is diagnostic, particularly when the anomalous ureter is dilated. The course of this ureter often may be followed down to and beyond the bladder.
- Diagnosis can be even more difficult when the kidney itself is ectopic. MR urography is indicated in the nonfunctioning kidney. Delayed contrast-enhanced CT with thin sections through the kidneys, coronal T1-weighted MRI, and MR urography are the most sensitive modalities for identifying an occult ectopic ureter.

Ureter, Neoplasm of

- Transitional cell carcinoma (TCC) accounts for about 93 % of ureteral neoplasms. Ureteral TCC, like bladder cancer, is more common in men than in women (male–female ratio,

2:1), and the incidence peaks in the seventh decade of life. TCCs of the ureter are most frequently found in the distal ureter (± 70 %).

- Upper tract TCCs are histologically and cytologically similar to bladder TCCs.
- Hematuria is present at diagnosis in 70–95 % of patients. Obstruction of the ureter or ureteropelvic junction due to a tumor mass causes flank pain in 8–40 % of cases. Other urinary tract symptoms, such as those associated with bladder irritation, and constitutional symptoms occur in less than 10 % of cases. The physical examination is usually unremarkable. In rare cases, a flank mass, caused either by the tumor or associated hydronephrosis, may be palpated.
- Hydroureteronephrosis is a common finding in CT. In some cases, the tumor can manifest as a mass of solid tissue (≥ 5 cm) with an attenuation value above urine in baseline images or more commonly as a filling defect or wall thickening in the excretory phase. Other useful CT findings for the identification of ureteric tumors are eccentric or concentric thickening of the ureteric walls, lumen stricture, and invasion of the adjacent structures (wall thickening and enhancement together with periureteric fat stranding are especially indicative of extramural tumor spread).
- On MR urography, the lesion appears as an intraluminal filling defect (with consequent dilatation of the collecting system proximally) or nonobstructive. This is useful in differential diagnosis with obstructive calculi. In addition, TCC typically appears as an irregular intraluminal defect, whereas a calculus displays regular and well-defined margins. The differential diagnosis between a tumor and a small stone can nonetheless be challenging. In baseline sequences indeed, TCC has signal intensity similar to that of the psoas muscle in T1-weighted images and slightly higher in T2. In this case, paramagnetic contrast medium, which should produce at least slight enhancement of TCC, is not always helpful.

Ureteral Bud, Atresia of

- Atresia of the ureteral bud at or below the ureteropelvic junction results in a severely dysplastic, nonfunctioning, cystic kidney.
- The diagnosis is usually easily established on the basis of characteristic imaging findings at ultrasound and renal diuretic or cortical scintigraphy of a nonfunctioning kidney that is replaced by multiple noncommunicating cysts with no residual normal-appearing parenchyma.
- At CT and MRI, the kidney is shown to be entirely replaced by multiple cysts of different sizes that are separated by a small amount of nonfunctioning, dysplastic parenchyma. In most patients with a multicystic dysplastic kidney, the fluid within the cysts is gradually absorbed and the kidney progressively decreases in size until it is no longer identifiable at ultrasound. In patients who have severe hypertension or other signs or symptoms suggestive of an occult, dysplastic kidney, MRI has been used to identify the tiny offending dysplastic remnant.

Urinoma

- Continued leakage of urine from the collecting system in the presence of urinary obstruction may lead to an encapsulated retroperitoneal urine collection called a urinoma. Urinomas may be associated with ureteropelvic junction obstruction; retroperitoneal fibrosis; retroperitoneal malignancy; cancer of the renal pelvis, ureter, or bladder; and a variety of conditions that cause bladder outlet obstruction. Urinomas may also occur in patients who have experienced blunt or penetrating abdominal trauma, renal surgery, or percutaneous procedure.

- Most urinomas leak into a subcapsular location or into the perirenal space within the Gerota's fascia. Urinomas may be confined, encapsulated fluid collections or may manifest as free fluid. Most urinomas occur posterior to the kidney, which is displaced upward anteriorly and sometimes laterally.
- Urinomas usually contain fluid of uniform water density. Intraperitoneal urine leaks are usually a result of penetrating or iatrogenic injury. Hydronephrosis is usually present and is aggravated by ureteric compression due to the urinoma. The nature of a urinoma may be confirmed by contrast-enhanced CT, which sometimes shows layering of contrast medium in the dependent part of the collection.

Urachal Anomalies

- Embryologically, the anterior bladder wall and umbilicus communicate with each other via a tubular channel (i.e., the urachus) which closes before birth. Failed obliteration of the urachal lumen results in four major types of anomalies: (1) the patent urachus, a persistent fistula between the bladder and umbilicus; (2) the urachal sinus, persistence of the urachus at its umbilical end; (3) the urachal diverticulum, persistence of the urachus at its bladder end; and (4) the urachal cyst, an encapsulation of fluid within a portion of the urachus that is closed at both the cranial and caudal ends. While the first two are best evaluated by fistulography, the other two can be easily identified by CT being both closed fluid-filled spaces.
- Urachal cysts account for 30 % of all urachal anomalies and primarily occur in the lower one-third of the urachus. They do not communicate with the bladder or umbilicus. The urachal cyst appears as a midline thin-walled, fluid-filled mass beneath the rectus abdominis muscle. Increased attenuation

or heterogeneous contents and wall thickening may be seen with infection or hemorrhage. Additional findings of pyourachus include bladder wall thickening, increased attenuation of the subcutaneous or mesenteric fat, rectus muscle thickening, intraperitoneal abscess, and a small amount of ascites.

- CT: The urachal diverticulum has a wide communication with the bladder dome and empties when the bladder is emptied.
- Benign urachal neoplasms including adenomas, fibromas, fibroadenomas, fibromyomas, and hamartomas are extremely rare; however, they are important in that they mimic urachal malignancy.

Ureteropelvic Junction Anomalies

- Anomalies of the ureteropelvic junction become manifest in conditions of hydronephrosis, i.e., with a more or less marked degree of dilatation of the pelvis and the calyces and the possible progressive compression of the renal parenchyma.
- The causes of hydronephrosis can be divided into primary (intrinsic and extrinsic) and secondary. The primary causes, which are very rare, include anomalies of the wall of the ureteropelvic junction and/or the ureters, such as ureteric constriction or hypoplasia, polyps, papillomas, valves, persistent fetal folds, and high insertion of the ureter. The most common extrinsic cause is the presence of an anomalous vessel on the lower pole which causes an obstruction, which in most cases is intermittent and is defined as intermittent ureteropelvic junction obstruction. This form accounts for around 20 % of cases of hydronephrosis involving ureteropelvic junction alterations. The secondary forms are generally related to high-grade vesicoureteric reflux. The consequent tortuous course of the ureter can cause a proximal obstruction. There are often associated malformations of other organ systems.

- Today, children affected by this condition are diagnosed asymptomatic, i.e., at prenatal US, whereas in the past, hydronephrosis was diagnosed late, often due to the presence of an abdominal mass or the onset of symptoms, such as fever, hematuria with or without renal colic, growth disorders, vomit, dyspepsia, and recurrent abdominal pain.
- Color Doppler ultrasound can identify the presence of an anomalous vessel. MR imaging is the preferred method because it is able to fully visualize the malformed urinary tract. Unenhanced heavily T2-weighted images and contrast-enhanced T1-weighted sequences can be applied to image the urinary tract. Premedication with furosemide (1 mg/kg) enables the upper urinary tract to be distended and the concentration of the paramagnetic contrast medium to be diluted.

Urolithiasis and Ureter Obstruction

- Renal calculi can be multiple, but in 80 % of cases, they are unilateral. Many patients will be affected by multiple stones throughout their lifetime, with estimated recurrence rates of 50 % within 5–10 years and 75 % within 20 years. The calculus, depending on the size, can migrate along the ureter until the diameter becomes too narrow for them to pass, thus causing urinary stasis and classic colicky pain.
- Most stones are passed spontaneously without causing any symptoms, especially if they are small with smooth walls. Renal colic is an excruciating and relentless pain with sudden onset. It often arises in the lumbar region and radiates with the classic loin-to-groin presentation. The pain may be associated with nausea and vomiting, intestinal gas, constipation and diarrhea, malaise, and lethargy.
- Non-contrast CT is the gold standard for the evaluation of urinary stone disease. It can detect both stones and urinary

tract obstruction thereby replacing radiography and excretory urography.

- CT can be performed rapidly, does not require the administration of contrast material, and is highly sensitive for the detection of stones of all sizes. Thin reconstructed sections (1–3 mm) are recommended for the detection of stones. The specificity of CT is nearly 100 %; thus, a positive study confirms the diagnosis of nephrolithiasis and patients should be treated appropriately.
- Intravenous contrast material administration is not routinely required for the diagnosis of calculi at CT. An important exception is nephrolithiasis secondary to HIV protease inhibitors, primarily indinavir. These stones are not radiopaque and signs of obstruction may be minimal or absent; thus, the diagnosis may be missed with ultrasound and non-contrasted CT scan.
- A possible pitfall of CT in patients who do not have evidence of urinary tract obstruction is the occasional inability to distinguish ureteral stones from phleboliths overlying the course of the ureter. This difficulty may be obviated by finding a "rim" sign on CT scanning due to circumferential edema from ureteral lithiasis.
- CT can be used to estimate stone burden, stone fragility, and stone composition.
- MRI is rarely used during the management of stone disease, except in the evaluation of pregnant patients, because this modality is not optimal for identifying stones. Thus, this modality can be utilized if there is a specific indication to reduce radiation exposure.

Uterine Adenomyosis

- Adenomyosis is a common gynecologic condition that affects menstruating women. The prevalence of adenomyosis is high in the female population (19–31 % of women).

- Adenomyosis is pathologically characterized by benign invasion of ectopic endometrium into the myometrium with adjacent smooth muscle hyperplasia.
- Although adenomyosis is not usually symptomatic, it is sometimes associated with menorrhagia, dysmenorrhea, and abnormal uterine bleeding.
- The lesion has low signal intensity on MR images because of the whorled hypertrophy of the myometrial smooth muscle which occurs around the glands. High-signal-intensity foci appearing within the nodules on T2-weighted images represent the glandular epithelium. These are occasionally hemorrhagic.

Uterine Sarcomas

- In addition to arising from the endometrium, uterine malignancies may originate from endometrial stroma (stromal sarcoma), pluripotent mesoderm (Mullerian mixed mesodermal tumors), and myometrial smooth muscle (leiomyosarcomas).
- Unlike endometrial carcinoma, mesenchymal malignancies often remain undetected by screening techniques and tend to be in an advanced stage at diagnosis. Spread by either the lymphatic or the hematogenous route is more likely at presentation compared with endometrial carcinoma.
- Uterine sarcomas represent only 1.3 % of myometrial tumors but are described as nonspecific heterogeneous solitary tumors with high vascularity. They are characterized by aggressive behavior and early dissemination.
- Mullerian mixed mesodermal tumors are aggressive malignancies with a propensity for advanced stage at diagnosis. Their biologic behavior and MRI characteristics are otherwise similar to those of endometrial carcinoma.

- Tumors derived from endometrial stromal tissues include benign stromal nodules, low-grade stromal sarcoma (indistinguishable from benign nodules but with lymphatic invasion), and endometrial stromal sarcoma. These tumors show intermediate to high signal intensity and infiltrate into the myometrium or vessels, an appearance dissimilar from that of leiomyomas.
- Ultrasonography is the first-line imaging technique for the detection of uterine myometrial tumors.

  MRI: Leiomyosarcomas arise from myometrial smooth muscle and usually occur in women between ages 40 and 60 years. Given the subtle difference between leiomyosarcomas and leiomyomas, it is unlikely that MRI will prove useful in differentiating between the two, although it serves to identify the myometrial origin of these tumors. Uterine sarcomas often manifest as a large myometrial mass with intermediate or high signal intensity on T2-weighted images, as do leiomyomas, which may be associated with various types of degeneration or cellular histological subtype, that could also mimic leiomyosarcoma. A large size at presentation and heterogeneously increased signal on T2-weighted images distinguish sarcomas from most, but certainly not all, leiomyomas.
- MRI may prove useful in the unusual venoinvasive form of this sarcoma (intravenous leiomyomatosis) to demonstrate the extent of intravascular disease.

Suggested Reading

Lawler LP, Jarret TW, Corl FM et al. 2005. Adult ureteropelvic junction obstruction: insights with three-dimensional multi-detector row CT. Radiographies; 25: 121–134

Berrocal T, López-Pereira P, Arjonilla A et al. 2002. Anomalies of the distal ureter, bladder. and urethra in children: embryologic, radiologic and pathologic features. Radiographies; 22: 1139–1164

Dueholm M, Lundorf E, Hansen ES et al. 2001. Magnetic resonance imaging and transvaginal ultrasonography for the diagnosis of adenomyosis. Fertil Steril; 76:588–594

Dalla Palma L, Pozzi-Mucelli R, Stacul F. 2001. Present-day imaging of patients with renal colic. Eur Radiol; 11:4–17

Teo SY, Babagbemi KT, Peters HE et al. 2008. Primary malignant mixed mullerian tumor of the uterus: findings on sonography, CT, and gadolinium-enhanced MRI. AJR Am J Roentgenol.;191: 278–83

Bass JE, Redwine MD, Kramer LA et al. 2000. Spectrum of congenital anomalies of the inferior vena cava: cross-sectional imaging findings. Radiographics; 20: 639–52.

V

Vulvar Cancer

- Vulvar carcinoma is a rare disease, which predominantly involves older women.
- The prognosis of vulvar carcinoma is related to the extent of the primary tumor and lymph node involvement.
- Squamous cell carcinoma accounts for approximately 80–90 % of vaginal malignancies.
- The main risk factor is infection with human papillomavirus (HPV).
- A clear cell carcinoma of the vagina is a rare cancer and often linked to exposure to diethylstilbestrol (DES). These tumors range from polypoid to infiltrating. Imaging has a limited role in their diagnosis, but MR is useful in assessing spread.
- Primary vaginal clear cell carcinoma not associated with DES is very rare.

V. Panebianco, J.J. Fütterer, *MDCT and MRI in Genitourinary Imaging*, 153
A-Z Notes in Radiological Practice and Reporting,
DOI 10.1007/978-88-470-5705-0_22, © Springer-Verlag Italia 2015

Vaginal Sarcoma

- Vaginal sarcomas account for 2 % of vaginal malignancies.
- Vaginal rhabdomyosarcomas are found almost exclusively in young children.
- Vaginal leiomyosarcoma is the most common sarcoma in adolescents and women.
- MR imaging is limited in the evaluation, except in outlining surrounding anatomy.
- Ultrasonography reveals a solid, mostly hypoechoic tumor.
- An angiosarcoma infiltrates the surrounding soft tissues. These highly vascular tumors often are amenable to preoperative angiographic embolization.

Vaginal Carcinoma

- The current evidence suggests that infection with human papillomavirus (HPV) plays a role in cervical cancer. The HPV DNA is present in most cervical cancers.
- Imaging does not have a primary role in cervical carcinoma detection.
- Carcinomas in the ectocervix tend to be polypoid and extend into the vagina. Endocervical cancers, on the other hand, infiltrate adjacent soft tissues.
- CT: Computed tomography detects a cervical carcinoma as a soft tissue tumor either in the ecto- or endocervix. However, only larger tumors can be detected, and the features of the tumors cannot be distinguished. These tumors enhance less with contrast than do the surrounding soft tissues.
- MRI: MRI provides highly accurate information on the morphology and extent of the cervical carcinoma. MRI reveals a cervical tumor as isointense to muscle on T1- and hyperintense on T2-weighted MR images. Most tumors are better

defined on T2-weighted images, although smaller ones enhance with contrast and tend to be best seen postcontrast. Cervical tumors demonstrate early and prolonged enhancement compared with poor enhancement of the normal cervical stroma.

Vaginal Congenital Anomalies

- MRI is not routinely used in the diagnosis of congenital or acquired vaginal cysts.
- Congenital cysts include both Gartner's and Mullerian duct cysts.
- Gartner's duct cysts originate from mesonephric (Wolffian) duct remnants that fail to reabsorb. They typically appear as cystic lesions in the anterolateral wall of the vagina, with low signal intensity on T1-weighted imaging and high signal intensity on T2-weighted imaging. In case proteinaceous or hemorrhagic contents are present, the T1-weighted images may show intermediate to high signal intensity.
- Mullerian duct cysts represent the embryological remnants of the paramesonephric duct.
- Acquired cysts include both vaginal inclusion cyst and Bartholin cyst. The latter arises from the Bartholin glands situated in the posterolateral introitus medial to the labia minora.
- Vaginal obstruction results in hemato (metro)colpos or hydrocolpos. At times, the obstruction evolves into a large pelvic soft tissue tumor, evident both clinically and with imaging.
- Congenital vaginal septa may occur either in isolation or with other Mullerian duct anomalies of the uterus and cervix.
- Obstructions range from imperforate hymen to a vaginal septum.

- MRI of hematocolpos reveals a high signal intensity both on T1- and T2-weighted images (blood products) and helps establish whether the distention extends into the fallopian tubes.

Varicocele

- A varicocele is characterized by abnormal tortuosity and dilatation of the veins in the pampiniform plexus of the spermatic cord caused by reflux of blood in the internal spermatic or gonadal veins. It consists of either a single enlarged vein or several freely communicating veins containing incompetent valves.
- Scrotal ultrasonography is the modality of choice for evaluating varicocele.
- MRI: MRI of an intratesticular varicocele reveals a tortuous tubular structure of low signal intensity on both T1- and T2-weighted images; it has a similar signal intensity as the testicular parenchyma. The more common extratesticular varicoceles have a serpiginous course and have a varied signal intensity, depending on flow.

Vas Deferens

- Malformations of these structures consist of cysts, agenesis, and partial atresia; an occasional one is associated with renal agenesis.
- Congenital absence of the vas deferens can be either bilateral or unilateral.
- The absence of vas deferens is identified by CT or MR imaging.

Von Hipple–Lindau (Kidney)

- Von Hippel–Lindau disease is a hereditary cancer syndrome caused by mutations of the VHL tumor-suppressor gene, which is located on the short arm of chromosome 3.
- This autosomal dominant disease has age-related penetrance of close to 100 % at age 60 years. Affected individuals develop several diseases including kidney cysts and clear cell carcinomas.
- Renal cysts are often multifocal and bilateral and are predominantly cortical in location. They do not progress to renal failure.
- Multicentric renal cell carcinomas are common, at times bilaterally.

Suggested Reading

Pecorelli S. Revised FIGO staging for carcinoma of the vulva, cervix, and endometrium. Int J Gynecol Obstet 2009;105(2):103–4.

Griffin N, Grant LA, Sala E. Magnetic resonance imaging of vaginal and vulval pathology. Eur Radiol. 2008 Jun;18(6):1269–80.

Williams AD, Cousins C, Soutter WP, et al. 2001. Detection of pelvic lymph node metastases in gynecologic malignancy: a comparison of CT,MR imaging,and positron emission tomography.AJR;177:343–348

Woodward PJ, Schwab CM, Sesterhenn IA. 2003. From the archives of the AFIP: extratesticular scrotal masses: radiologic-pathologic correlation. Radiographics.;23(1):215–40.

Saleem SN. MR imaging diagnosis of uterovaginal anomalies: current state of the art. Radiographics. 2003;23(5):e13.

Ozsarlak O, Tjalma W, Schepens E, et al. 2003. The correlation of preoperative CT, MR imaging, and clinical staging (FIGO) with histopathology findings in primary cervical carcinoma. Eur Radiol;13:2338–235.

Vaganovs P, Bokums K, Miklaševics E, et al. 2013. Von Hippel-Lindau syndrome: diagnosis and management of hemangioblastoma and pheochromocytoma. Case Rep Urol.

W

No lemma

V. Panebianco, J.J. Fütterer, *MDCT and MRI in Genitourinary Imaging*,   159
A-Z Notes in Radiological Practice and Reporting,
DOI 10.1007/978-88-470-5705-0_23, © Springer-Verlag Italia 2015

X

Xanthogranulomatous Pyelonephritis (XGN)

- It is an uncommon condition characterized by chronic granulomatous process, induced by recurrent bacterial urinary tract infection, in which the renal parenchyma is ultimately replaced with lipid-laden (foamy) macrophages.
    Most patients are middle-aged and diabetic female patients who present with symptoms like flank pain, hematuria, malaise, weight loss, and low-grade fever.
- The preoperative diagnosis of XGN is difficult because of its nonspecific clinical presentation. Hematuria and hydronephrosis are sometimes encountered.
- CT: Typical findings are the combination of a nonfunctioning unilateral enlarged kidney and parenchymal inflammation. A central calculus within a contracted renal pelvis, multiple areas of low attenuation representing expansion of the calyces filled with pus, and inflammatory changes in the perinephric fat are often present. The walls of the dilated calyces demonstrate enhancement due to the vascularity of the surrounding granulation tissue and compressed normal renal parenchyma.

V. Panebianco, J.J. Fütterer, *MDCT and MRI in Genitourinary Imaging*,   161
A-Z Notes in Radiological Practice and Reporting,
DOI 10.1007/978-88-470-5705-0_24, © Springer-Verlag Italia 2015

- MRI: The morphologic features are similar for both CT and MRI. Signal intensity characteristics may vary. The solid mass demonstrates iso- to high signal intensity compared with the renal parenchyma on T1-weighted images. The signal intensity on T2-weighted images is isointense compared with the contralateral normal kidney. The fluid-filled expanded calyces demonstrate low signal intensity on T1-weighted images and high signal intensity on T2-weighted images. The perirenal infiltration shows low signal intensity on both T1- and T2-weighted images.

Suggested Reading

Craig WD, Wagner BJ, Travis MD. 2008. From the Archives of the AFIP Pyelonephritis: Radiologic-Pathologic Review, RadioGraphics 28: 255–276.

Goldman SM, Hartman DS, Fishman EK, Finizio JP, Gatewood OM, Siegelman SS. CT of Xanthogranulomatous pyelonephritis: Radiologic-pathologic correlation. AJR Am J Roentgenol 1984;141:963–9.

Claes H, Vcneecken R, Oyen R, Van Damme B. Xanthogranulomatous pyelonephnitis with emphasis on computerized tomography scan. Urology 1987;29:389–93.

Verswijvel G, Oyen R, Van Poppel H, Roskams T. Xanthogranulomatous pyelonephritis: MRI findings in the diffuse and the focal type. Eur Radiol. 2000;10(4):586–9.

Y

No lemma

V. Panebianco, J.J. Fütterer, *MDCT and MRI in Genitourinary Imaging*,   163
A-Z Notes in Radiological Practice and Reporting,
DOI 10.1007/978-88-470-5705-0_25, © Springer-Verlag Italia 2015

Z

No lemma

V. Panebianco, J.J. Fütterer, *MDCT and MRI in Genitourinary Imaging*, 165
A-Z Notes in Radiological Practice and Reporting,
DOI 10.1007/978-88-470-5705-0_26, © Springer-Verlag Italia 2015